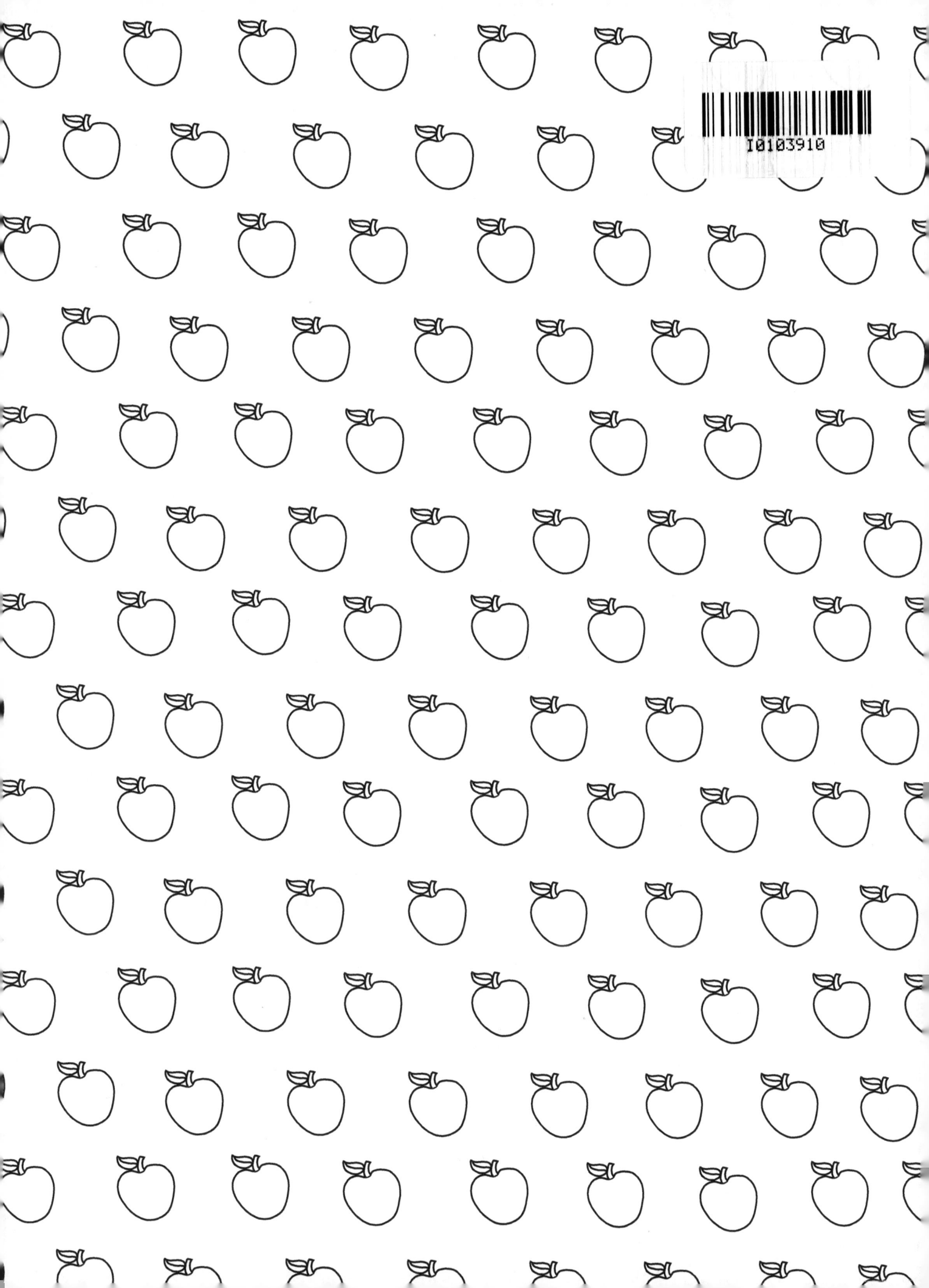

THE WONDERFUL WHOLEFOOD GARDEN

The Health Food Coloring Journey

Karen Martin

HeartAlignBooks

The Wonderful Wholefood Garden is a unique coloring in book that contains captivating and bedazzling illustrations, conveying the wild wonder and beauty of whole foods in practical and aesthetic combinations. Karen's intricate illustrations also contain a wonderful combination of creativity and scientific rigor. Watch the fruits and vegetables come to life as you learn about good health and get a dose of stress relief at the same time.

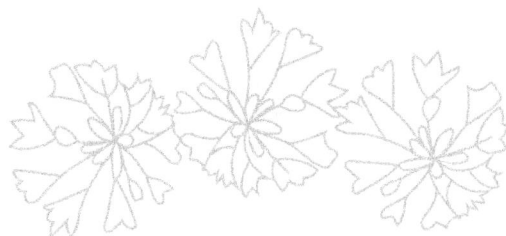

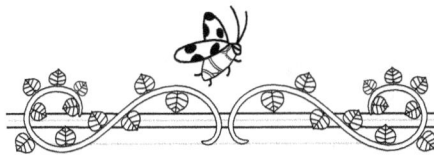

Follow me on a dance with romance
Discover natures gifts
and healing art
May wholefood love
fill your heart

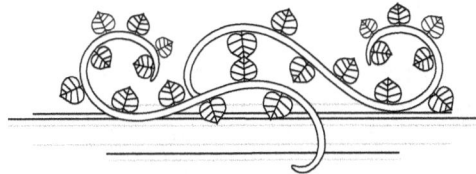

INTRODUCTION

Plant foods are full of vitamins, minerals, fats, protein, carbohydrates, dietary fiber, healthy gut bacteria, antioxidants and thousands of plant chemicals called phytonutrients or phytochemicals.

Phytonutrients are compounds that may aid in preventing cancer, diabetes, heart disease, vision loss, bad cholesterol and osteoporosis.

A major group of phytonutrients are antioxidants. Antioxidants neutralise oxidants, which are free radicals found in the environment and the body. Antioxidants help stop cell damage casued by oxidants and help prevent infections.

Flavonoids, carotenoids, triterpenoids and polyphenols are types of phytonutrients with antioxidant properties. Alpha-carotene and beta-carotene are pro-vitamin A carotenoids, because they can actually be converted to active vitamin A. Vitamin A is also an antioxidant too, along with Vitamin C and E (A-C-E!) and the minerals selenium and manganese.

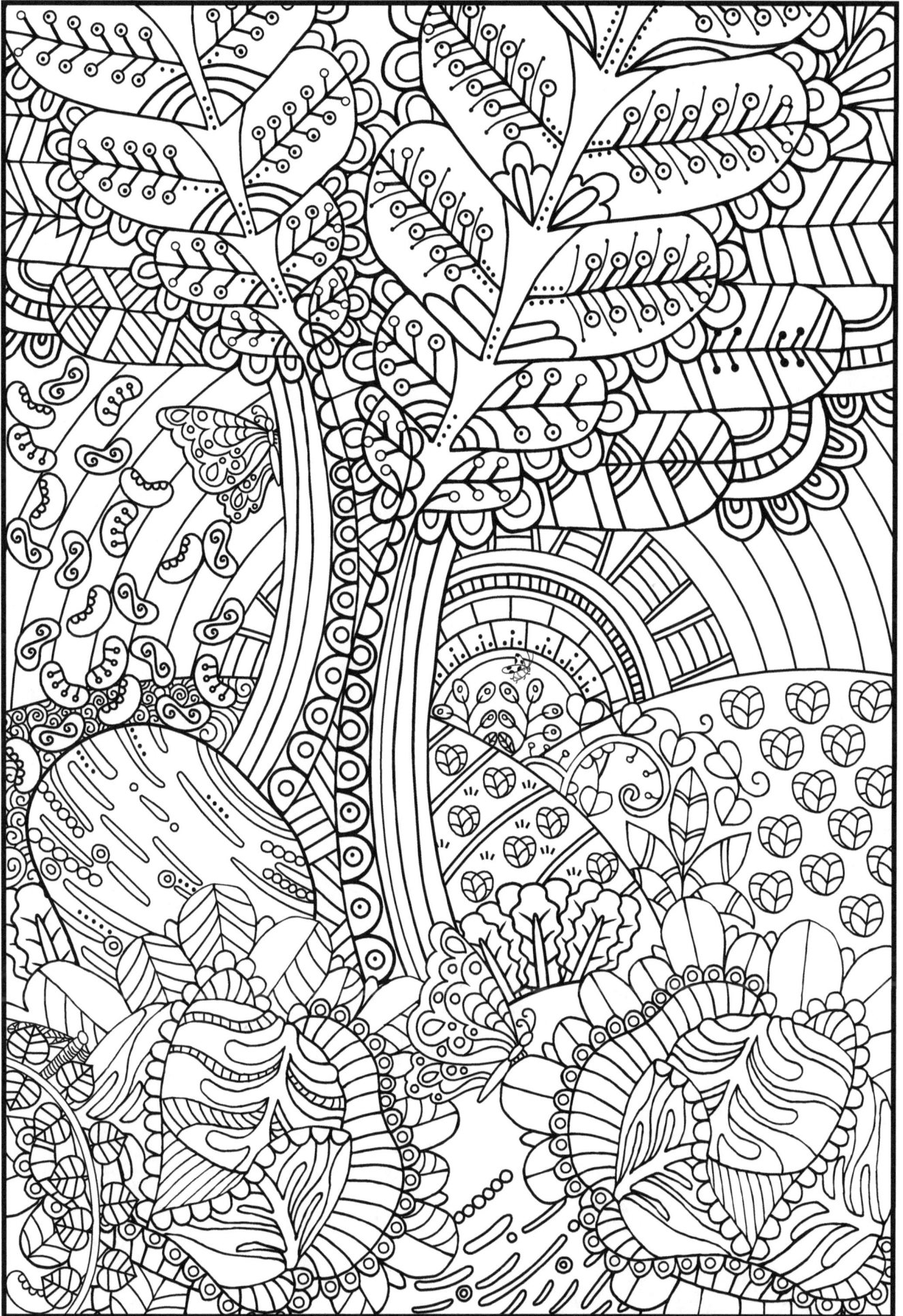

BERRIES

Berries are rich in catechin, a powerful polyphenol antioxidant that may help prevent Alzheimer's, cancer and heart disease. Catechin has anti-bacterial and anti-biotic properties. Berries contains the polyphenol flavonoid type plant pigment quercitin. Quercitin is a powerful antioxidant that is anti-inflammatory and anti-histamine and may help protect against allergies, cancer, heart disease, high cholesterol and rheumatoid arthritis.

OATS

Oats are a nutrient rich whole-grain.
Oats contain many antioxidants including avenanthramide,
which has anti-inflammatory and anti-histamine properties.
Oats may help lower blood pressure
and cholesterol levels.

BANANA

Bananas are full of vitamins and minerals including: niacin (B3),
pyridoxine (B6), folate (B9), calcium, iron, magnesium, manganese
and potassium. The high potassium in bananas helps regulate
blood pressure, heart beat and improve mental alertness.

LEAFY GREENS

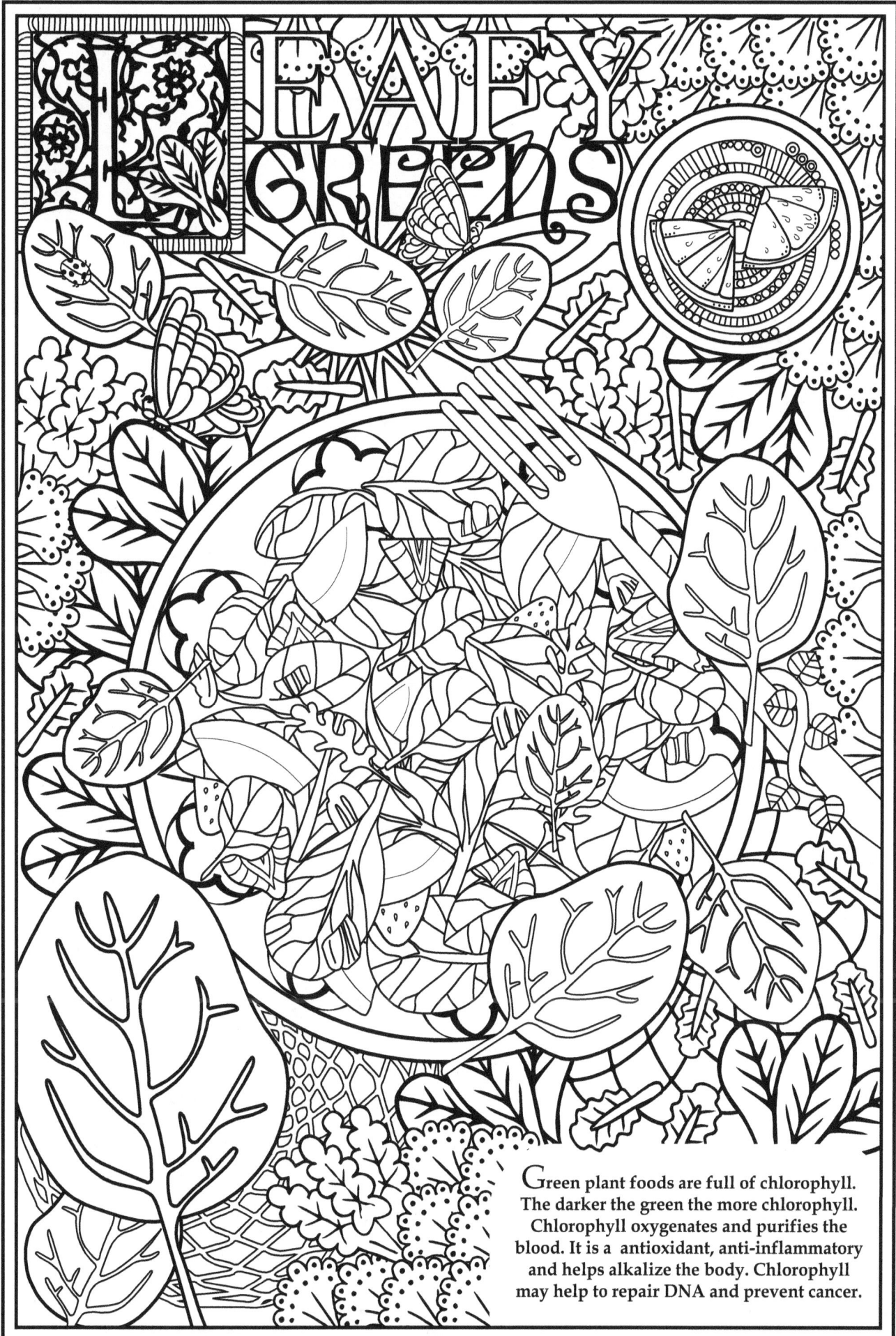

Green plant foods are full of chlorophyll. The darker the green the more chlorophyll. Chlorophyll oxygenates and purifies the blood. It is a antioxidant, anti-inflammatory and helps alkalize the body. Chlorophyll may help to repair DNA and prevent cancer.

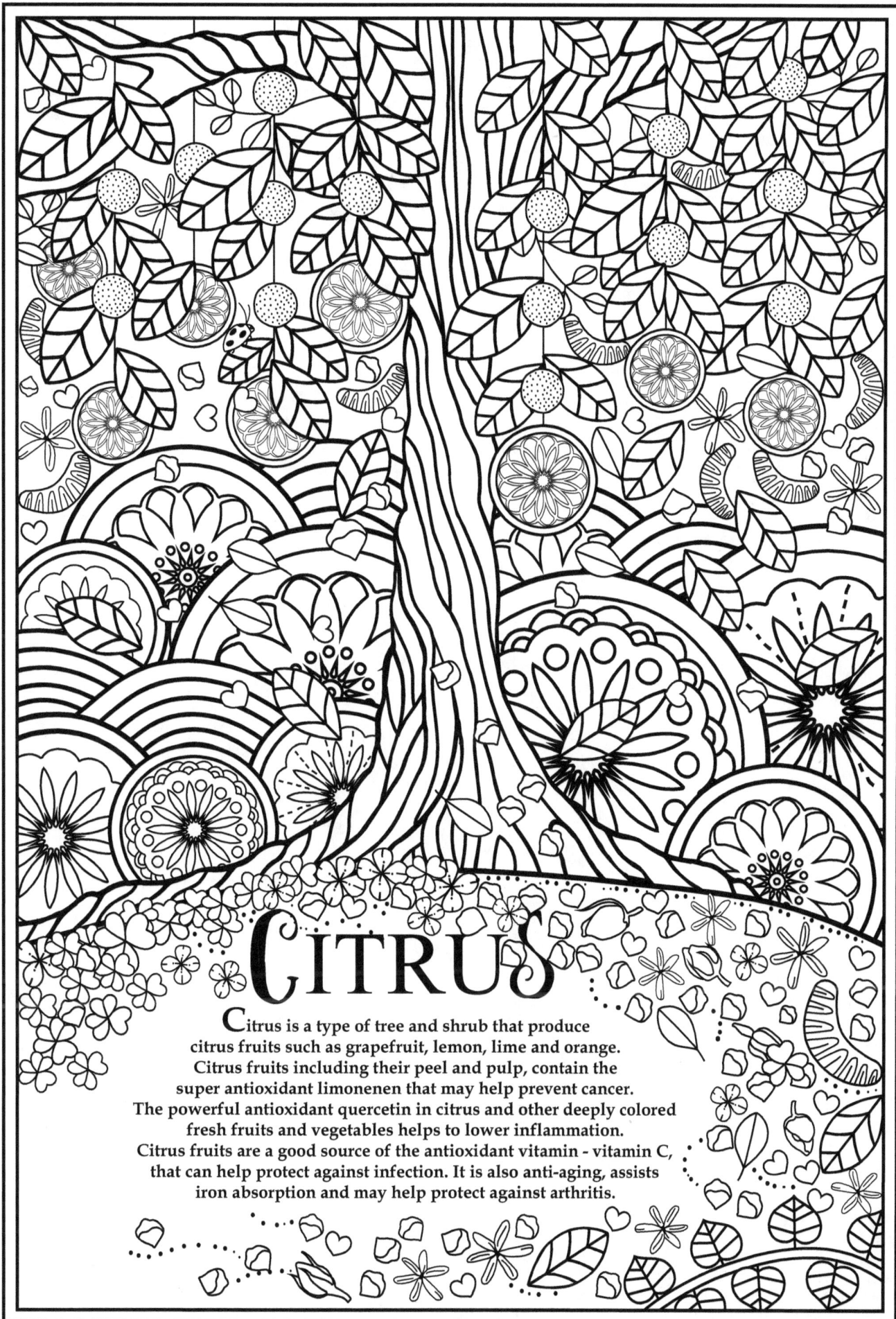

CITRUS

Citrus is a type of tree and shrub that produce
citrus fruits such as grapefruit, lemon, lime and orange.
Citrus fruits including their peel and pulp, contain the
super antioxidant limonenen that may help prevent cancer.
The powerful antioxidant quercetin in citrus and other deeply colored
fresh fruits and vegetables helps to lower inflammation.
Citrus fruits are a good source of the antioxidant vitamin - vitamin C,
that can help protect against infection. It is also anti-aging, assists
iron absorption and may help protect against arthritis.

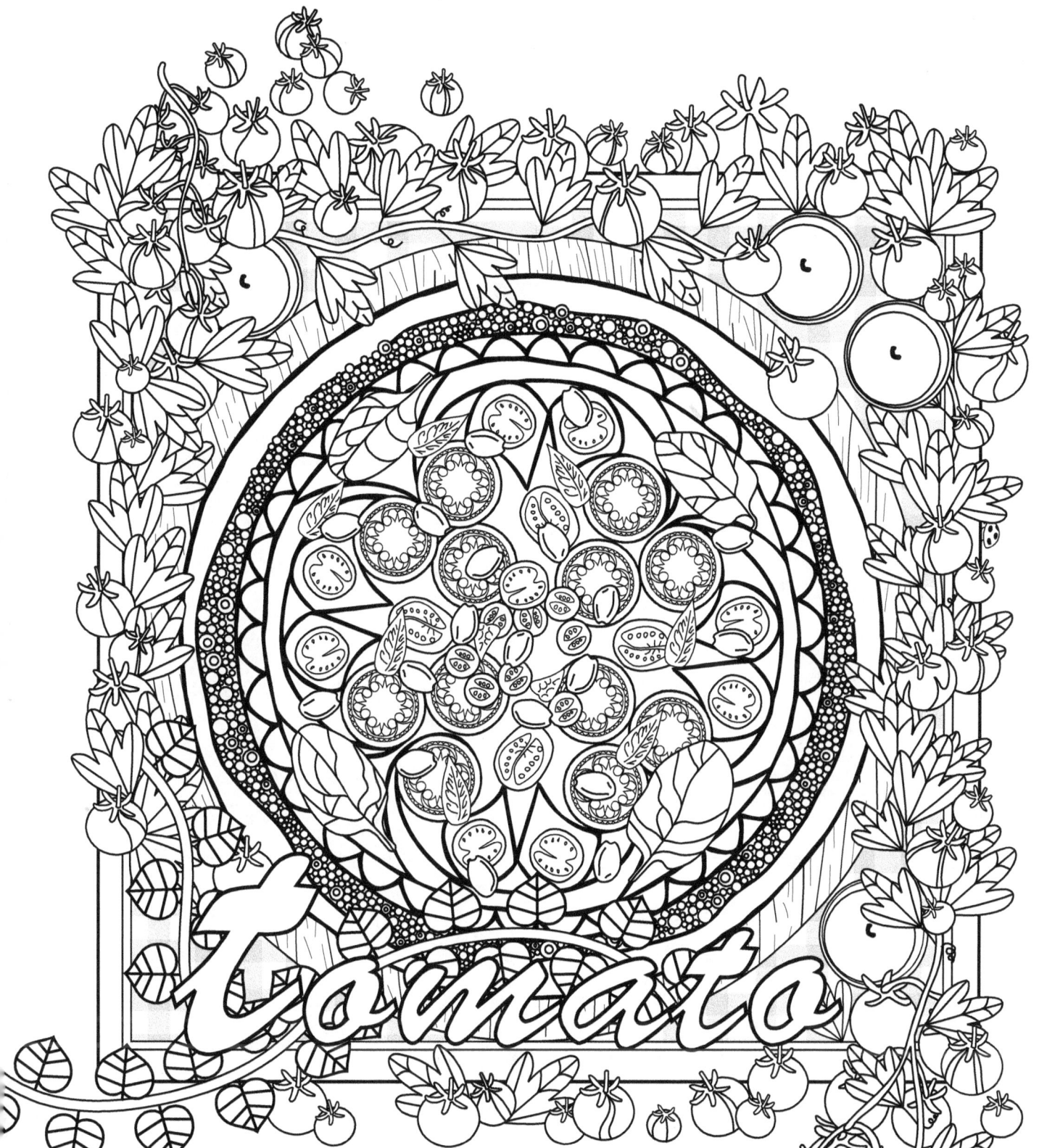

Tomatoes contain vitamins: biotin (B7), C, E, K and minerals: calcium, iodine, iron, phosphorus and potassium. Tomatoes are high in Vitamin E. Vitamin E helps blood circulation and is also an antioxidant. They contain lycopene, a powerful carotenoid antioxidant that gives tomatoes their red color. Lycopene can help protect your skin and bones and may help to prevent certain types of cancers.

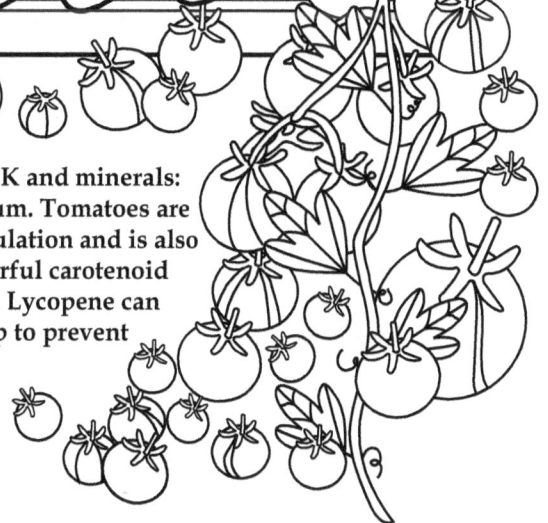

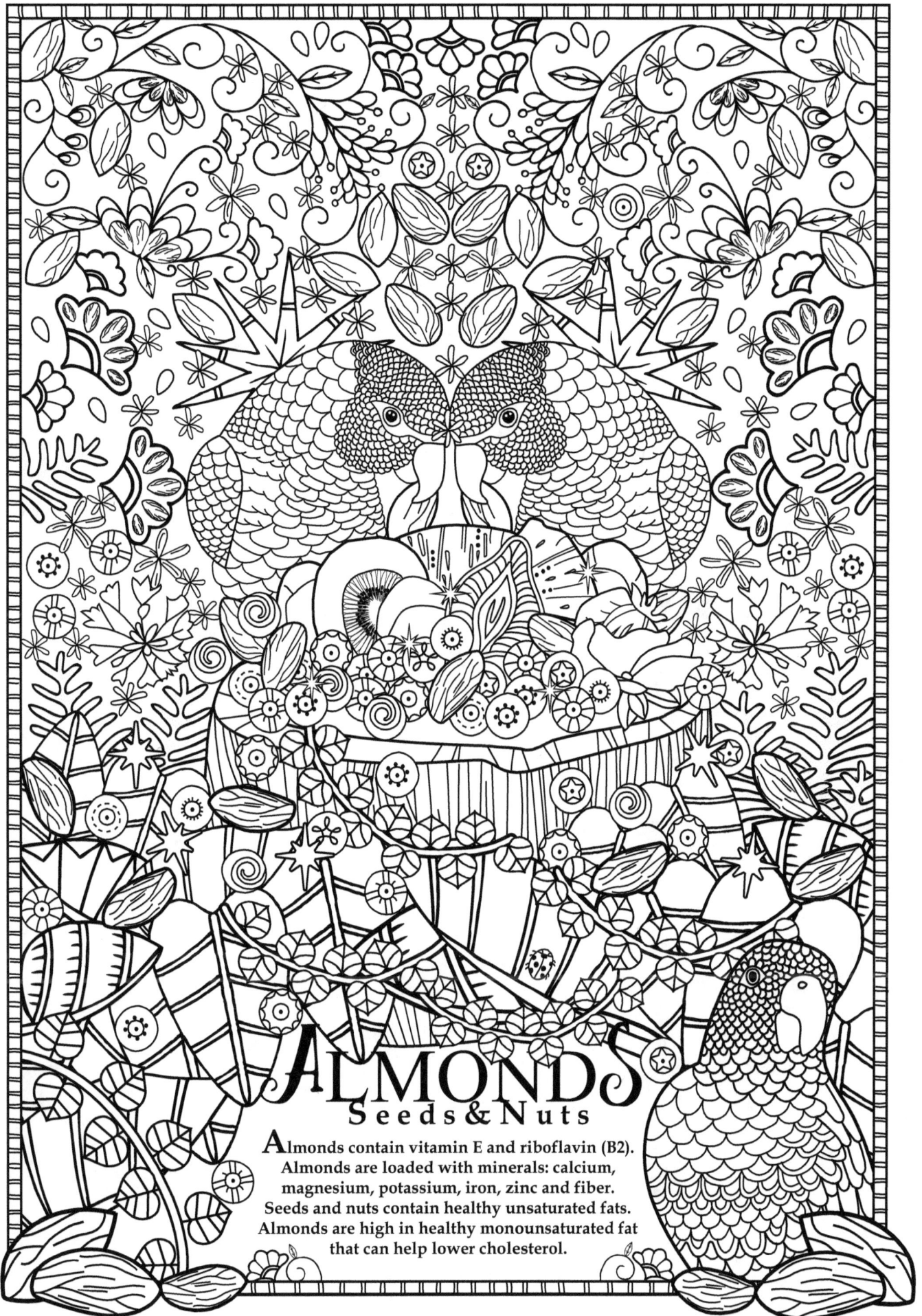

Almonds
Seeds & Nuts

Almonds contain vitamin E and riboflavin (B2).
Almonds are loaded with minerals: calcium,
magnesium, potassium, iron, zinc and fiber.
Seeds and nuts contain healthy unsaturated fats.
Almonds are high in healthy monounsaturated fat
that can help lower cholesterol.

WATERMELON

Watermelon contains vitamins; A, C, pyridoxine (B6) and mineral: magnesium and potassium. Watermelon is rich in flavonoids, carotenoids, triterpenoids and the amino acid citrulline that helps reduce fat in the fat cells. Watermelon contains the carotenoid antioxidant lycopene, associated with lowering the risk of certain types of cancers, as well as; high blood pressure, cholesterol, osteoporosis and age related macular degeneration.

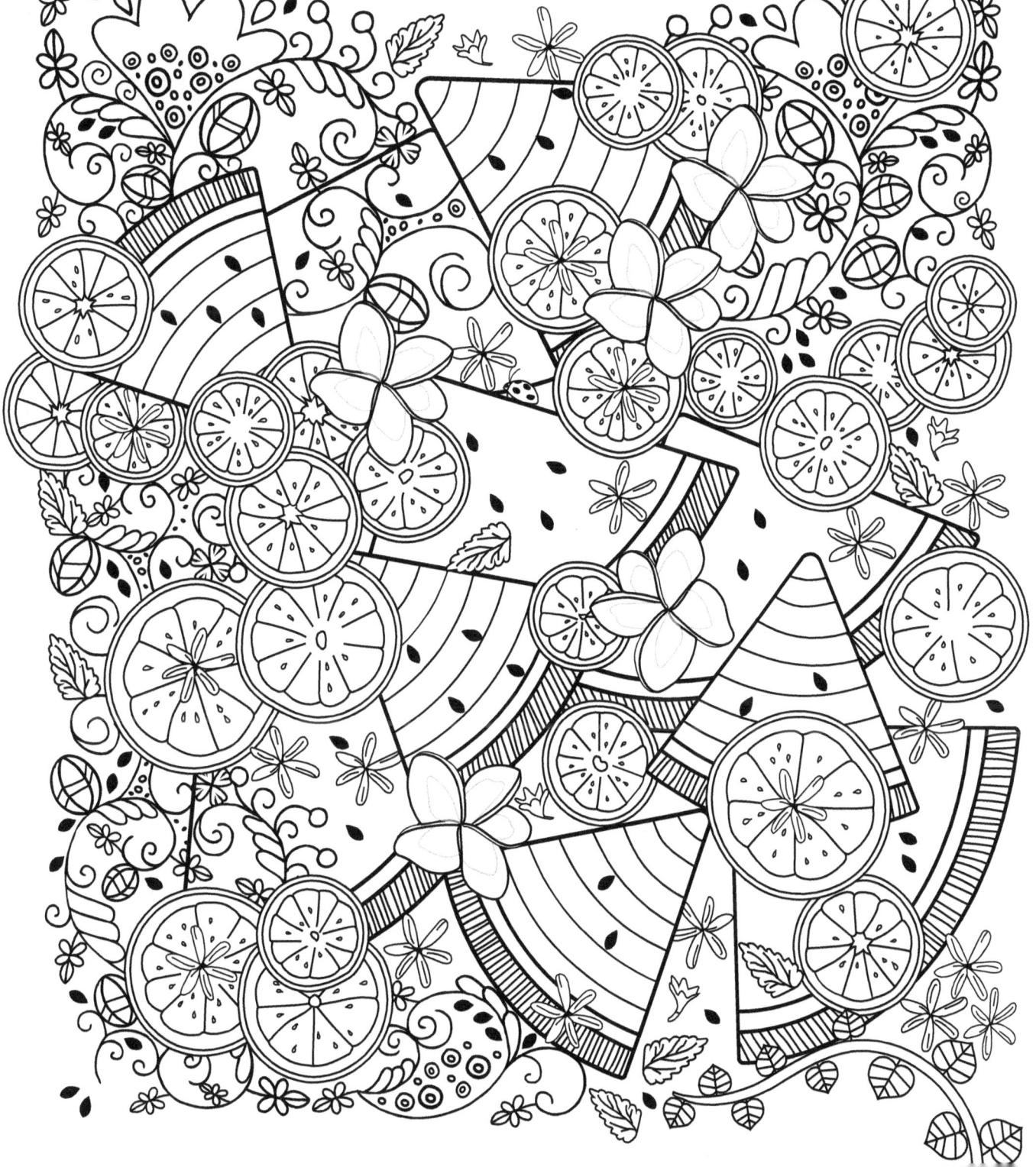

Apples contain malic and tartaric acids that inhibit "bad" bacteria in the gut. The pectin in apples is a soluble-fiber that can detox lead and mercury from the body. Triterpenoids, found in apple skin may have anti-cancer effects. Chlorogenic acid in apples may help lower blood pressure, activate weight loss, improve mood and reduce the risk of cancer and diabetes. Apples may help protect against heart disease, diabetes, Alzheimer's, asthma and cancer.

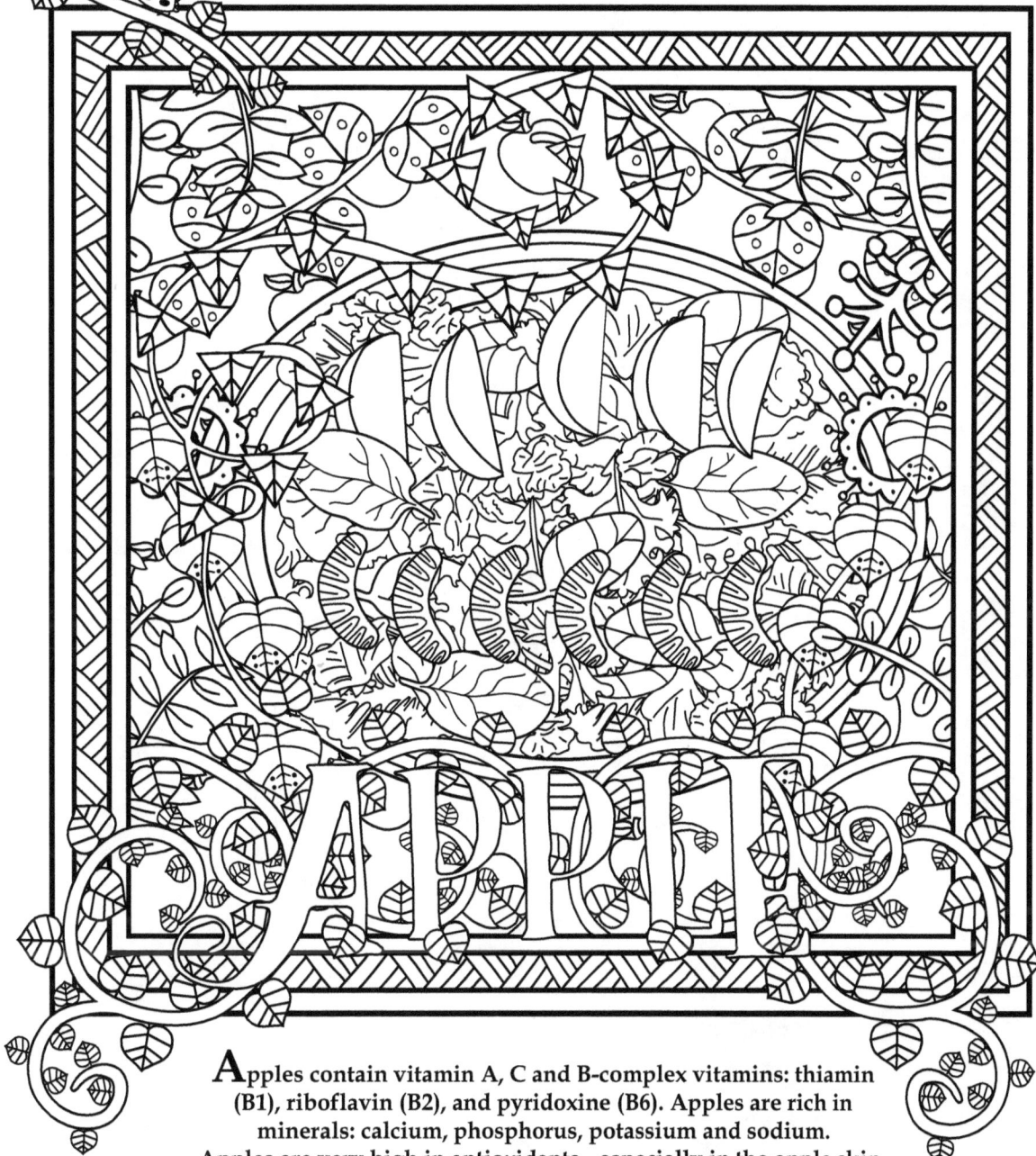

APPLE

Apples contain vitamin A, C and B-complex vitamins: thiamin (B1), riboflavin (B2), and pyridoxine (B6). Apples are rich in minerals: calcium, phosphorus, potassium and sodium. Apples are very high in antioxidants - especially in the apple skin. Apples are high in powerful flavonoid antioxidants such as: catechin, epicatechin, kaempferol, myricetin, phloridzin, procyanidins and quercetin.

CHERRIES

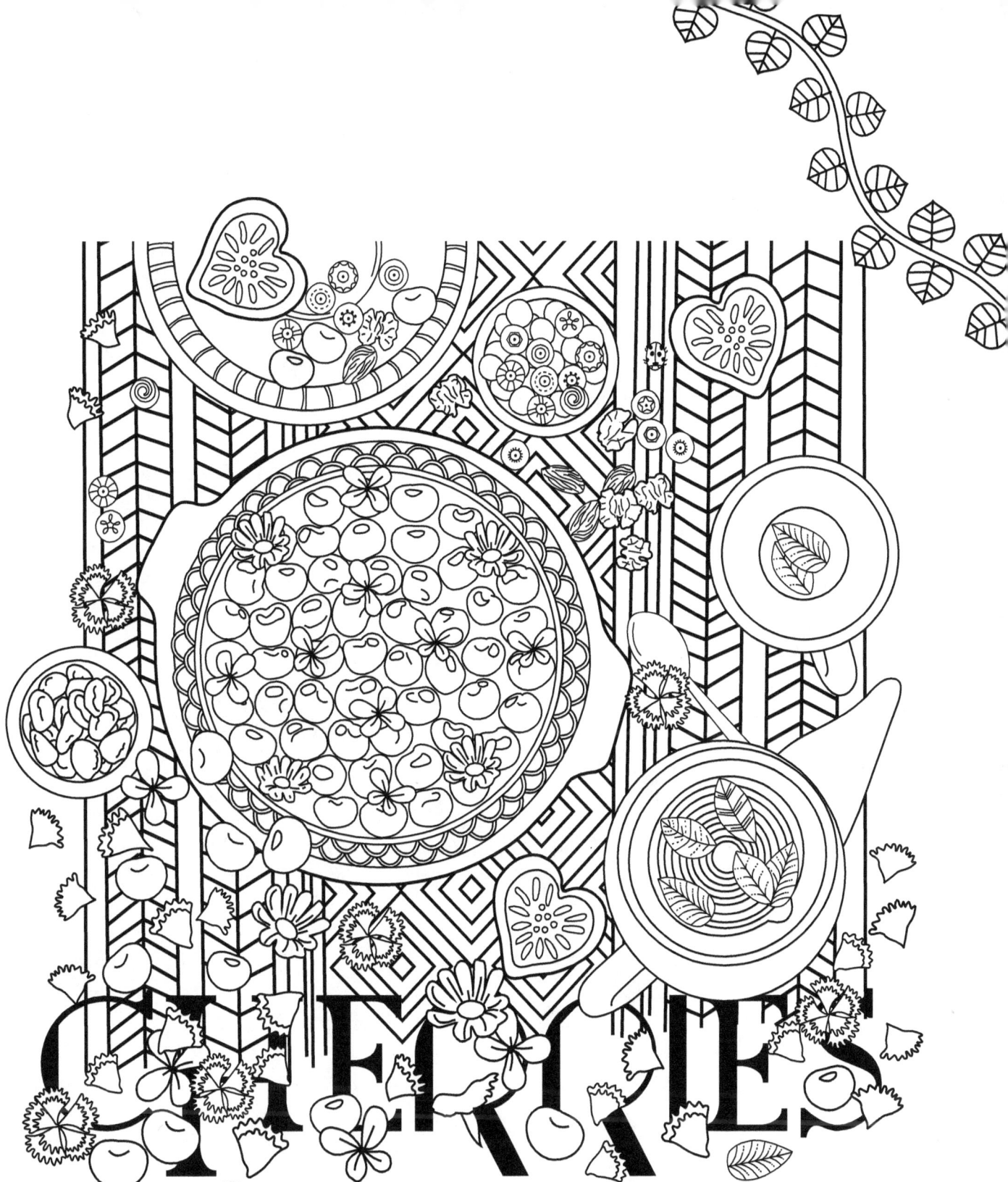

Cherries have the highest amount of antioxidants than any other fruit. The antioxidant anthocyanins give cherries their red color. Cherries contain vitamin A, calcium, folate, and potassium. The high levels of potassium mean that cherries help regulate blood pressure and heart rate. Cherries are anti-inflammatory and contain melatonin that helps to regulate sleep cycles.

Olives are a good source of Polyphenol antioxidants such as Hydroxytyrosol. Hydroxytyrosol has anti-inflammatory and antibacterial properties that may protect the heart, bone loss and help prevent cancer. The phenolic compound Oleocanthal in olives acts as a natural painkiller. Olive extracts are anti-allergic due to anti-histamine properties. Olives are unique due to their high source of anti-oxidants and anti-inflammatory properties, that may also help to protect against cancer.

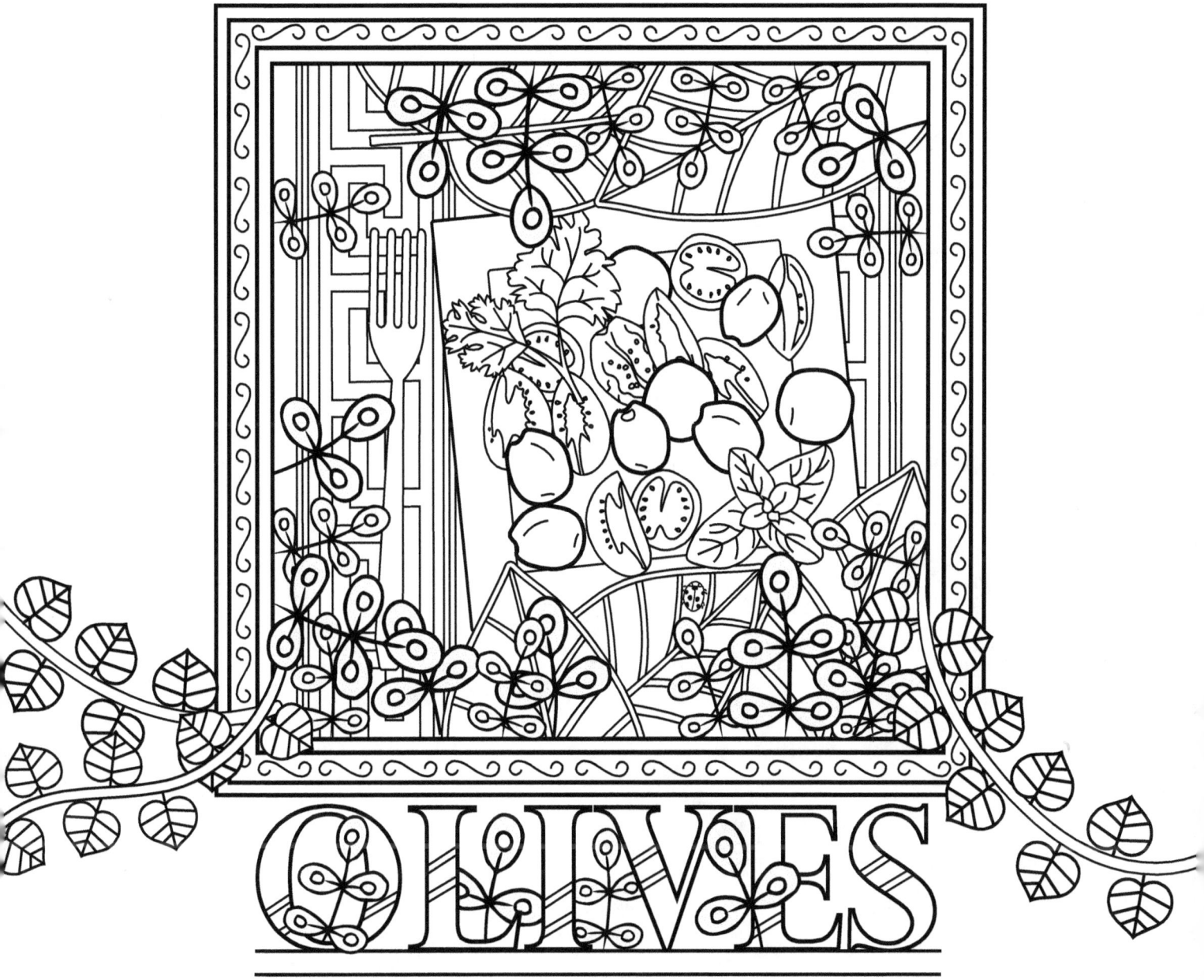

OLIVES

Olives are stone fruits, that are high in the antioxidant Vitamin E. Olives contain beta-carotene (Vitamin A), K, E, calcium, copper, iron and sodium. They contain oleic acid - monounsaturated fats (healthy fat) that helps promote heart health and healthy skin. Olives are rich in many phytonutrients including: hydroxytyrosol, kaempferol, luteolin, oleonolic acid, oleuropein, tyrosol, and quercetin.

BELL PEPPERS

Bell Peppers (also known as capsicums) are high in vitamin A and C, folate (B9)
and potassium. Folate may help to prevent Alzheimer's and certain cancers.
The potassium in bell peppers helps blood flow to the brain.
Bell Peppers grow from green to yellow to red.
Red Bell Peppers contain the most folate (B9) and potassium.

MUSHROOM

Mushrooms contain vitamin C, riboflavin (B2), niacin (B3) and minerals:
copper, iron, phosphorus and potassium. Mushrooms also contain the antioxidant trace mineral selenium. Selenium may help lower the risk of certain
cancers. Mushrooms can also contain vitamin D when exposed to sunlight.

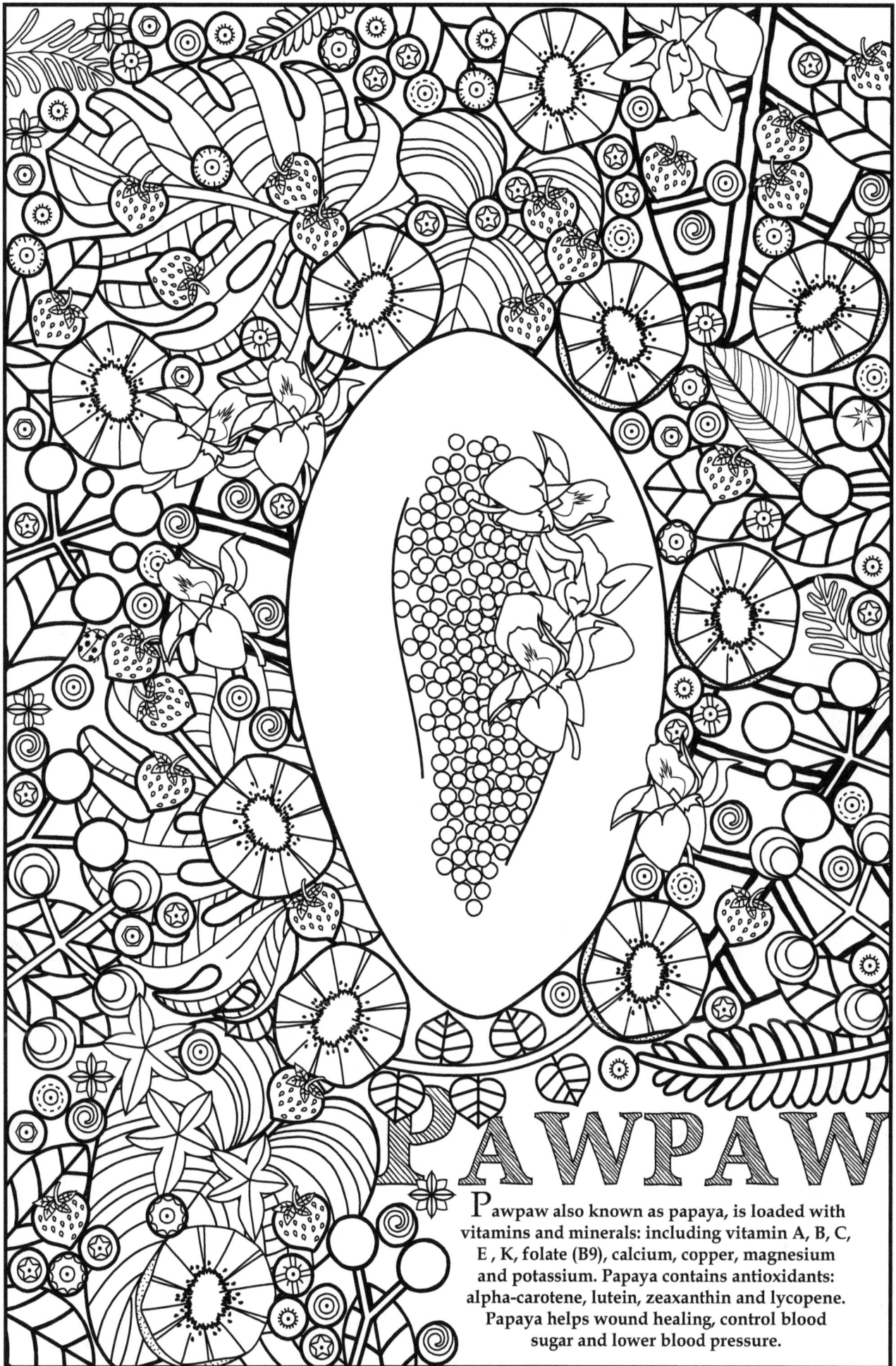

PAWPAW

Pawpaw also known as papaya, is loaded with vitamins and minerals: including vitamin A, B, C, E , K, folate (B9), calcium, copper, magnesium and potassium. Papaya contains antioxidants: alpha-carotene, lutein, zeaxanthin and lycopene. Papaya helps wound healing, control blood sugar and lower blood pressure.

Carrots contain carotenoids: alpha-carotene, lutein and lycopene. That supports the immune system including: eye, heart and bone health and may prevent disease including certain cancers. Other powerful phytonutrients in carrots include anthocyanins and polyacetylenes that may also have anti-cancer properties.

CARROT

Carrots are very high in beta-carotene (that converts to Vitamin A). Carrots contain vitamins: pyridoxide (B6) and biotin (B7) and small amounts of almost every essential vitamin. They are a rich source of vitamin C, which stimulates the activity of white blood cells for a healthy immune system.

CELERY

Celery contains a unique enzyme called molybdenum that helps metabolise toxins from the body and may help lower the risk of cancer. Celery is anti-bacterial and anti-inflammatory. Celery supports liver health. Protects the digestive tract from ulcers, reduces blood pressure and protects against heart disease.

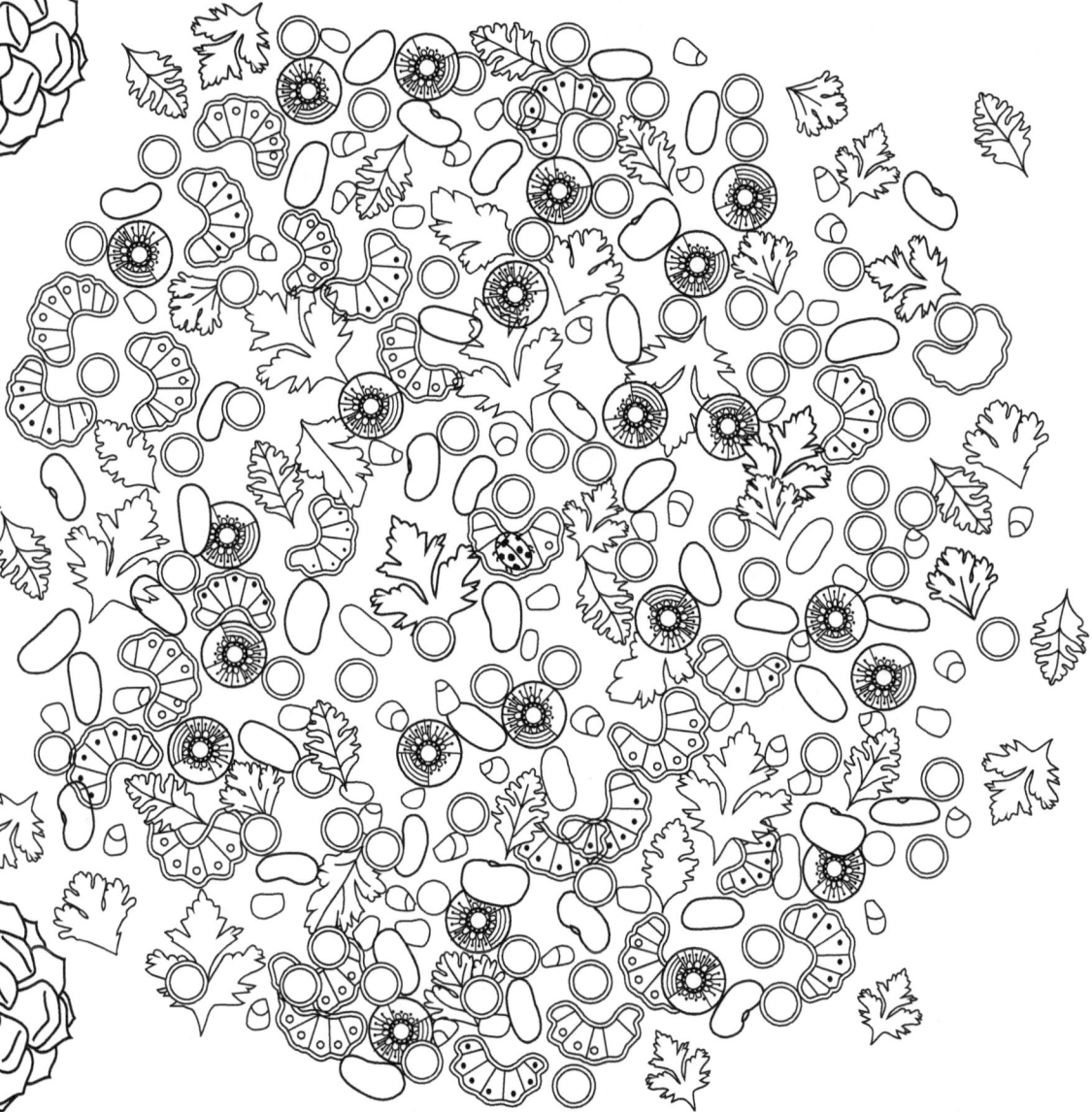

Celery contains vitamin A, riboflavin (B2), pyridoxine (B6), folate (B9), K and minerals: calcium, copper, magnesium, phosphorus and potassium. Celery contains many different kinds of phenolic, flavanoid types of antioxidants including lutelin. Lutelin may help protect the eyes and the brain from inflammation and Neuro-degenerative disease.

ROSEMARY

Rosemary is high in carnosic acid, that may help enhance learning and spatial memory. The phytonutrients in rosemary may help protect against Alzheimer's and other neuro degenerative diseases.

PARSLEY

Parsley is a herb rich in antioxidants: beta carotene and lutelin. Lutelin has anti-cancer qualities and helps protect the brain. Parsley is high in the blood purifier chlorophyll.

BASIL

contains an impressive source of nutrients including beta-carotene (Vitamin A), pyridoxine (B6), folate (B9), vitamin C and K, calcium, copper, iron, magnesium, manganese, potassium and omega-3 fatty acids. Basil also contains many phytochemicals: flavonoids, carotenoids, coumarin, anthhocyanins and essential oils.

Pineapple is high in B group vitamins: thiamin (B1), pantothenic acid (B5), pyridoxine (B6), folate (B9): vitamin C and minerals: copper, magnesium, manganese and potassium. Pineapple contains many polyphenol antioxidants including flavonoids and phenolic acids.

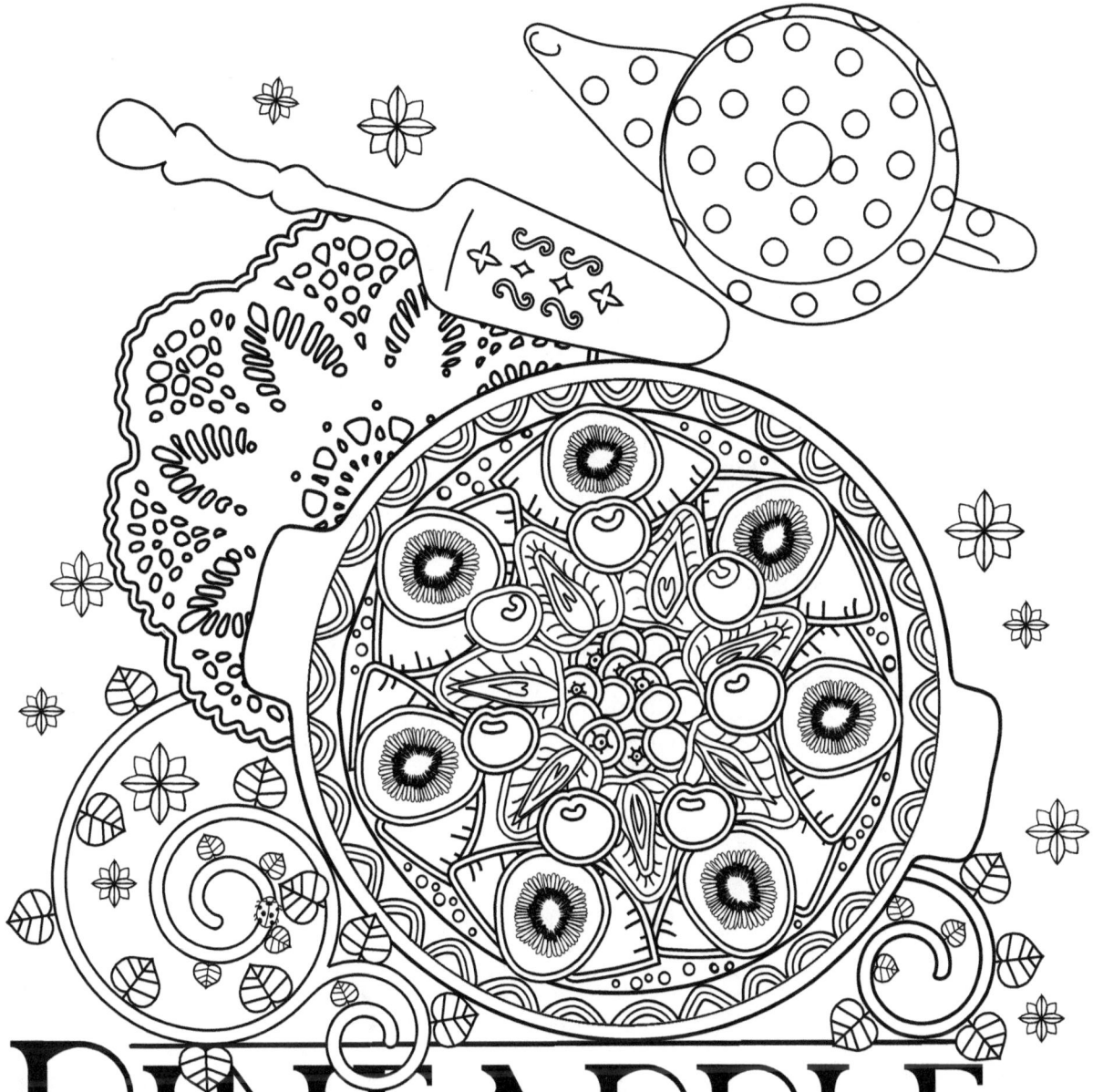

PINEAPPLE

Pinapple is actually a group of berries that have fused together to from a collective fruit. Pinapple contains the unique anti-inflammatory enzyme called bromelain. Bromelain breaks down proteins in your mouth reducing respiratory and sinus congestion. Bromelain can fight bacteria and infections. Pineapples are an excellent source of fibre and can help strengthen the gums.

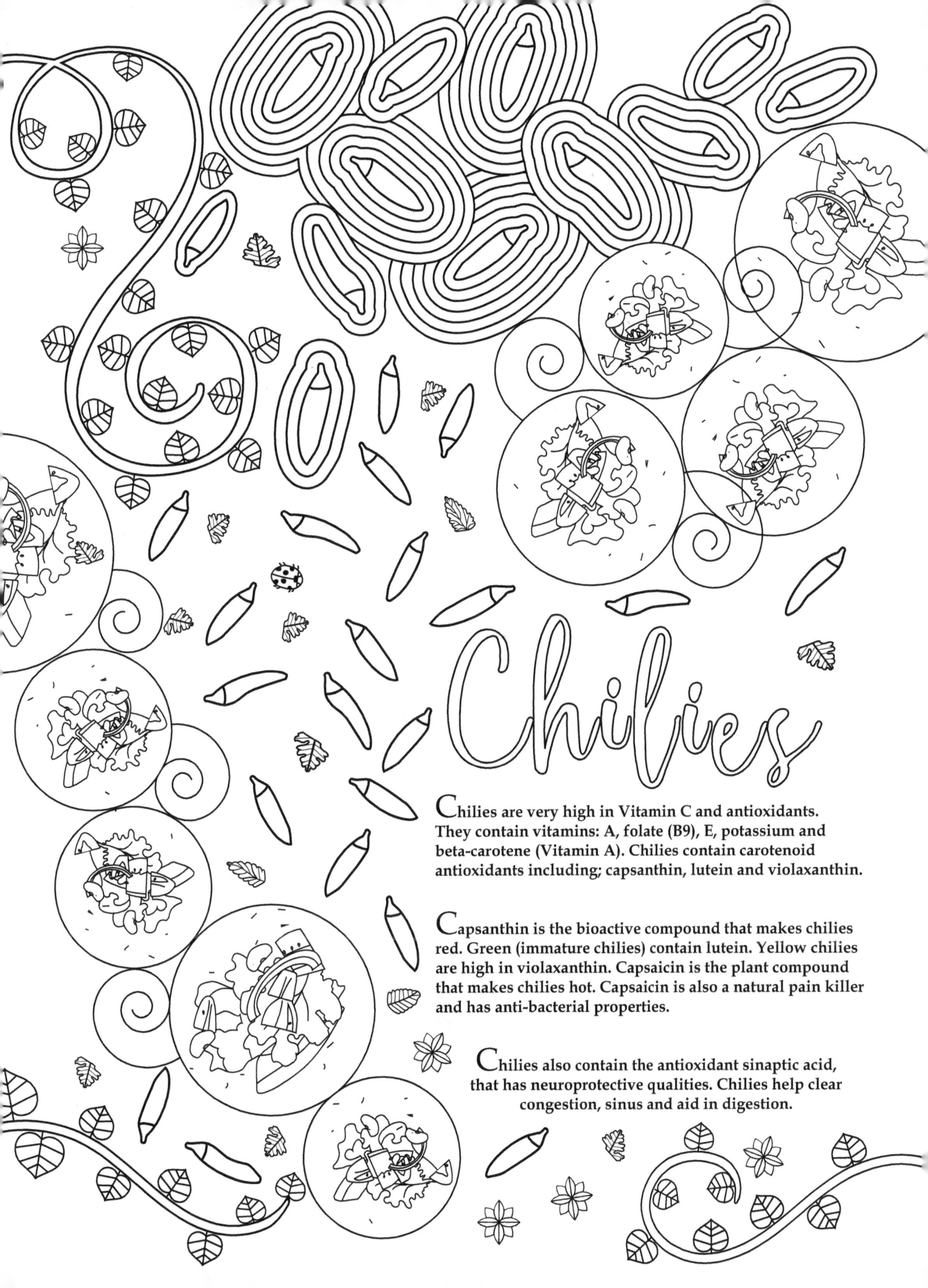

Chilies

Chilies are very high in Vitamin C and antioxidants. They contain vitamins: A, folate (B9), E, potassium and beta-carotene (Vitamin A). Chilies contain carotenoid antioxidants including; capsanthin, lutein and violaxanthin.

Capsanthin is the bioactive compound that makes chilies red. Green (immature chilies) contain lutein. Yellow chilies are high in violaxanthin. Capsaicin is the plant compound that makes chilies hot. Capsaicin is also a natural pain killer and has anti-bacterial properties.

Chilies also contain the antioxidant sinaptic acid, that has neuroprotective qualities. Chilies help clear congestion, sinus and aid in digestion.

KIWIFRUIT

Kiwi fruit contains vitamin: A, pyridoxine (B6), cobalamin (B12), E, calcium, iron, magnesium, potassium, omega-3 fatty acids and dietary fiber. Kiwi fruit contains many antioxidants and is exceptionally high in the antioxidant vitamin C. The high vitamin C may reduce inflammation and symptoms associated with asthma.

The vibrant green in kiwi fruit are due to carotenoids and chlorophyll. Kiwis are alkaline promoting, helping to restore blood to normal pH balance. Carotenoids in kiwi fruit include: beta-carotene, lutein and xanthophylls. Kiwi fruit contains phenolic compounds: flavonoids and anthocyanins. The enzyme actinidain in kiwi fruit helps digestion, as it breaks down protein. The serotonin in Kiwi fruit helps to improve mood and sleep quality.

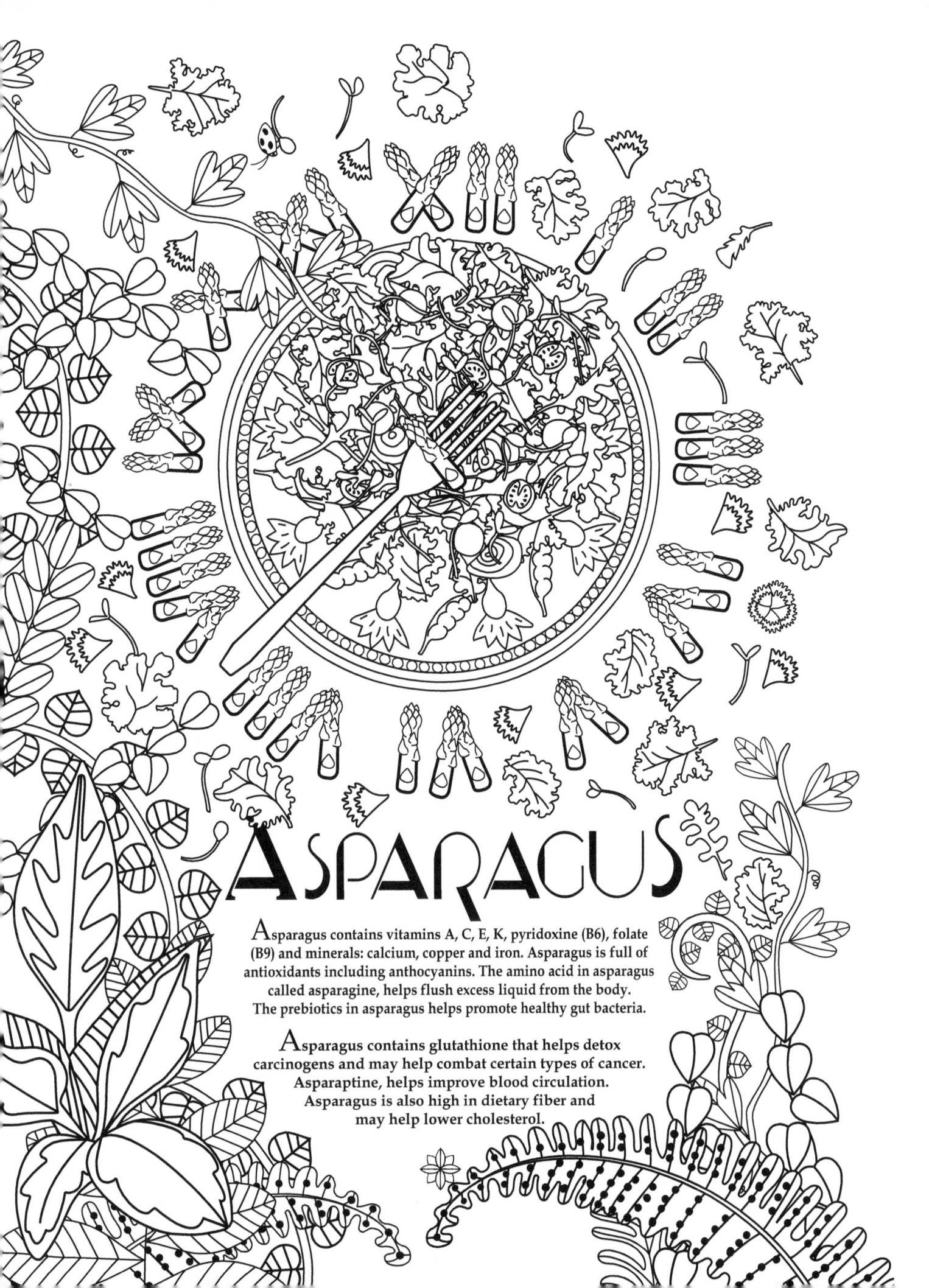

ASPARAGUS

Asparagus contains vitamins A, C, E, K, pyridoxine (B6), folate (B9) and minerals: calcium, copper and iron. Asparagus is full of antioxidants including anthocyanins. The amino acid in asparagus called asparagine, helps flush excess liquid from the body. The prebiotics in asparagus helps promote healthy gut bacteria.

Asparagus contains glutathione that helps detox carcinogens and may help combat certain types of cancer. Asparaptine, helps improve blood circulation. Asparagus is also high in dietary fiber and may help lower cholesterol.

Mango

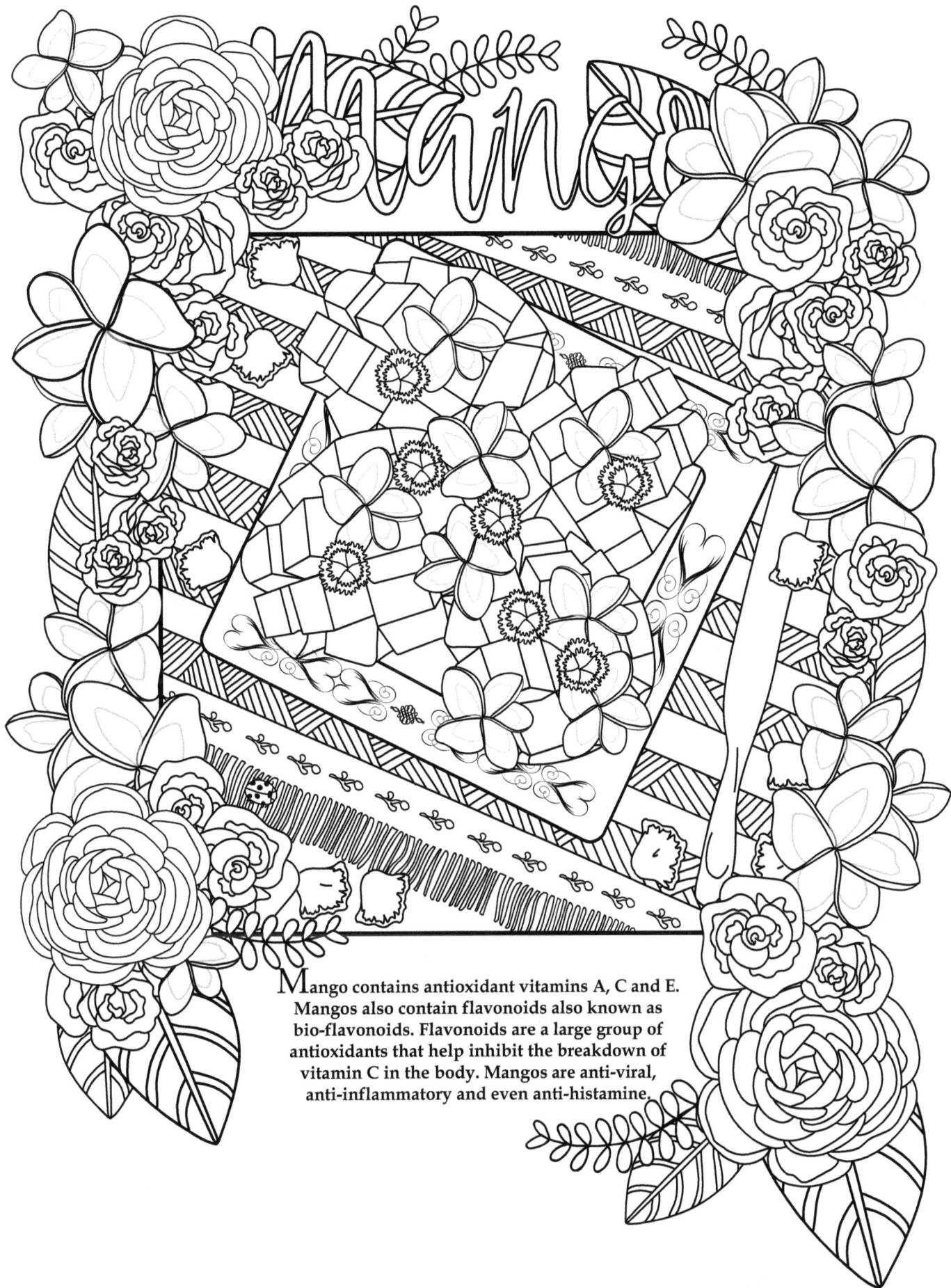

Mango contains antioxidant vitamins A, C and E. Mangos also contain flavonoids also known as bio-flavonoids. Flavonoids are a large group of antioxidants that help inhibit the breakdown of vitamin C in the body. Mangos are anti-viral, anti-inflammatory and even anti-histamine.

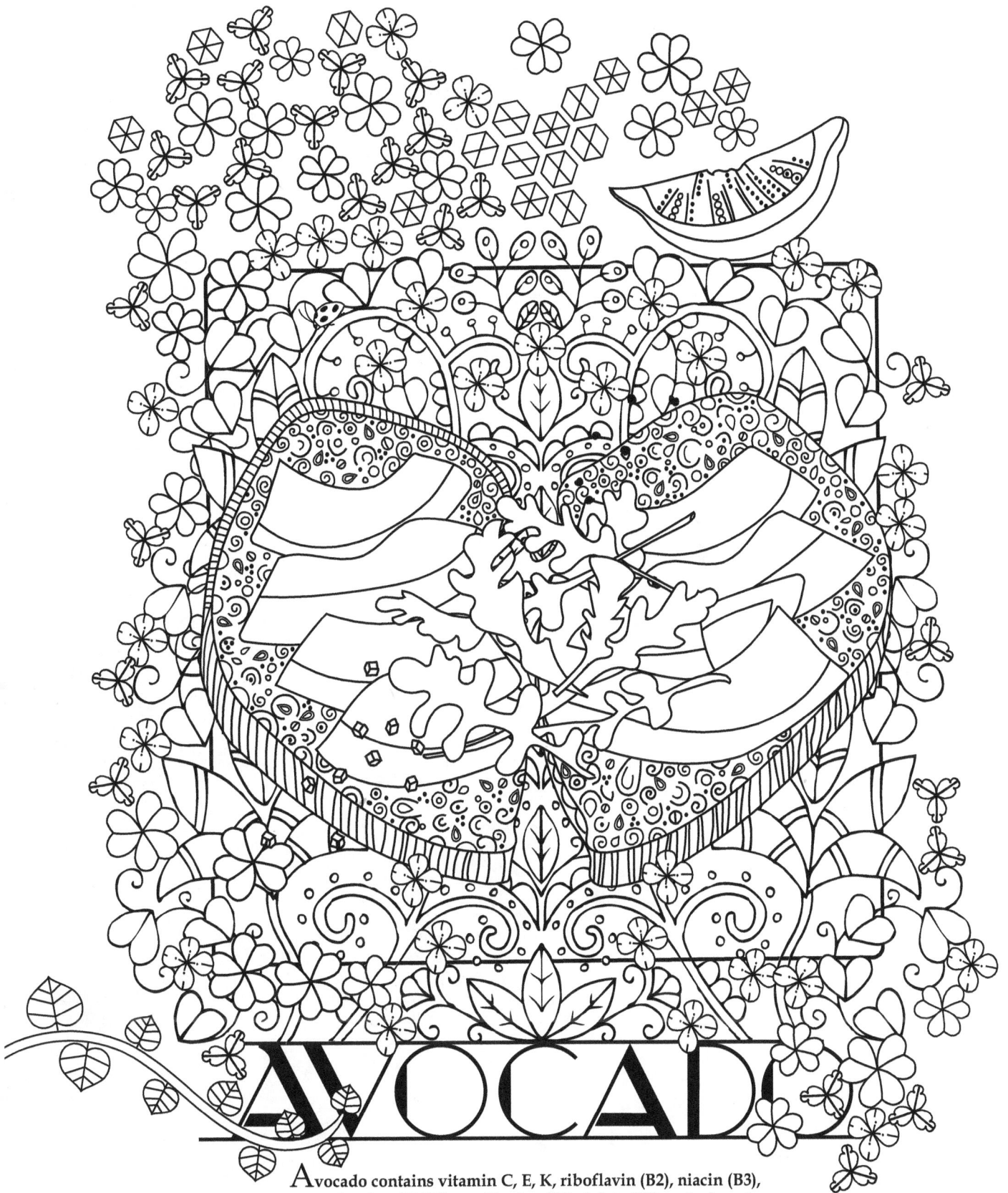

AVOCADO

Avocado contains vitamin C, E, K, riboflavin (B2), niacin (B3), panto-thenic acid (B5), pyridoxine (B6), folate (B9) and minerals: magnesium and potassium. They are full of healthy, monounsaturated fats and are an excellent source of omega-3 fatty acids. Avo's are full of antioxidants: alpha-carotene, beta-carotene, beta-cryptoxanthin, lutein and zeaxanthin. They are anti-inflammatory and also help to regulate hormones.

BEETROOT

Beetroot contains vitamins: A, C and folate (B9) and is rich in many minerals including: calcium, copper, iron, maganese, mangnesium, phosphorus, potassium, selenium, sodium and zinc.

Beets contains unique phytonutrients such as betaine, that may prevent liver disease, and betalain, that may help prevent some cancers. Beetroot also contains nitrate that may help lower blood pressure and help to prevent dementia.

KALE

Kale is a green leafy vegetable containing
vitamins A, B (B1, B2 , B3) and C.
Kale is full of minerals that rhyme with yum
calcium, magnesium, potassium and sodium.

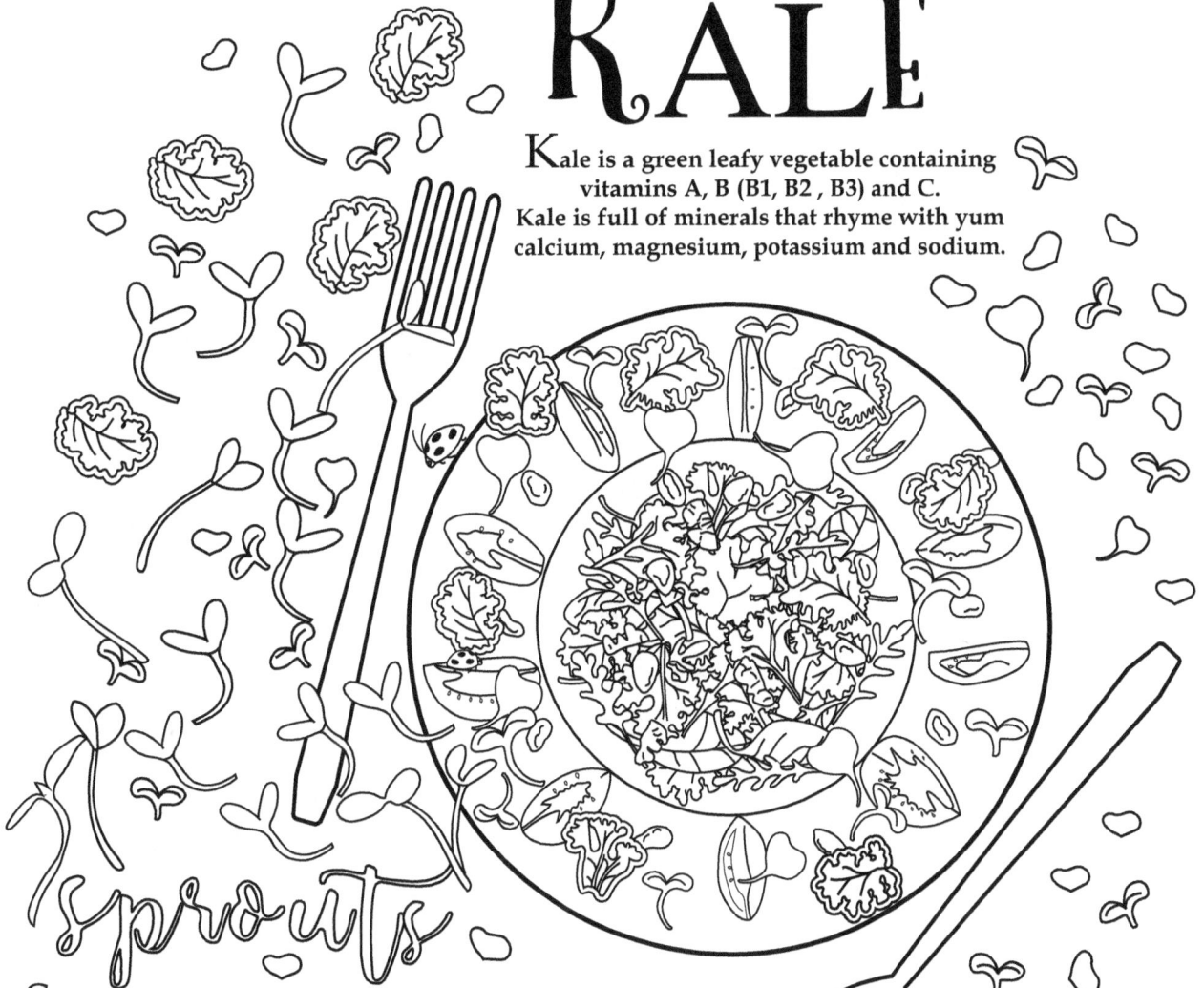

sprouts

Sprouts contain a super concentration of nutrients.
Sprouts have similar benefiets to seeds.
The process of sprouting brings out many enzymes.

SPINACH

Spinach contains the powerful antioxidant beta-carotene. Spinach is high in vitamin
niacin (B3) and contains vitamins A, C, E, K, pyridoxine (B6) and folate (B9).
Spinach is full of minerals: calcium, copper, iron, maganese, magnesium, phosphorus,
potassium, sulphur and is rich in zinc. Spinach contains the antioxidant chlorophyll,
a green pigment found in all green plants, that has anti-cancer effects.

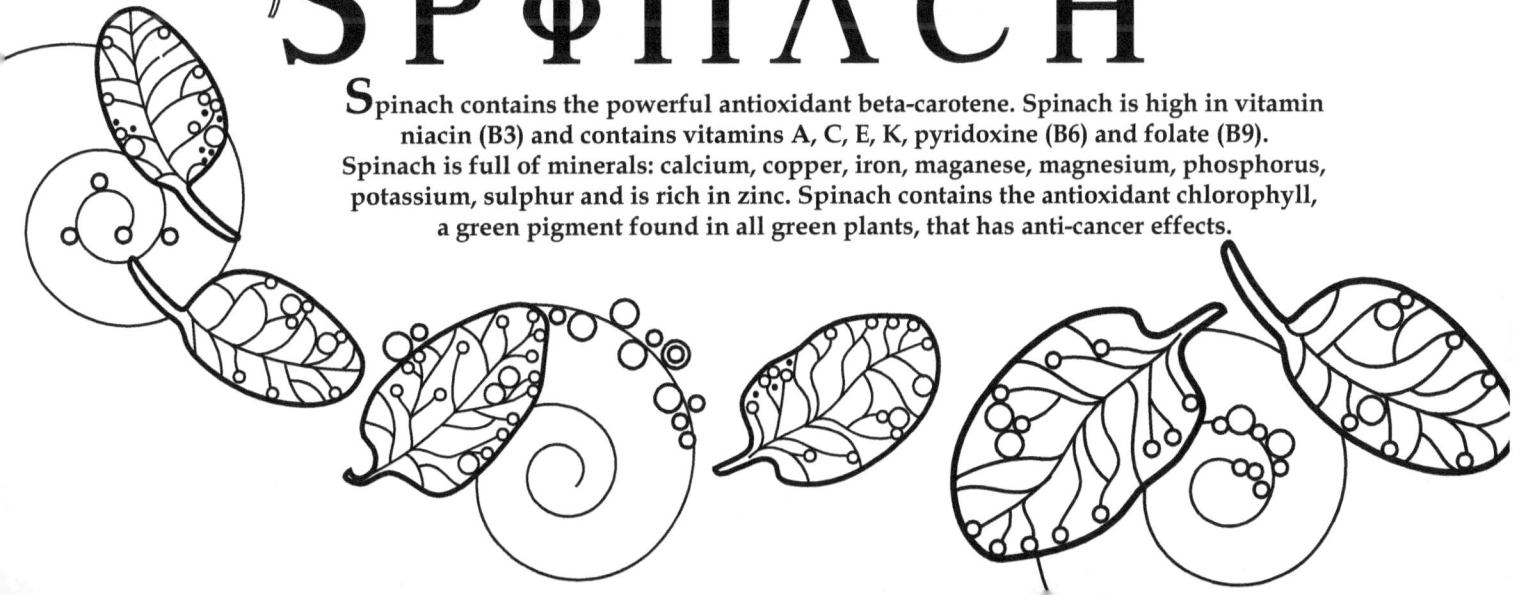

Pumpkin

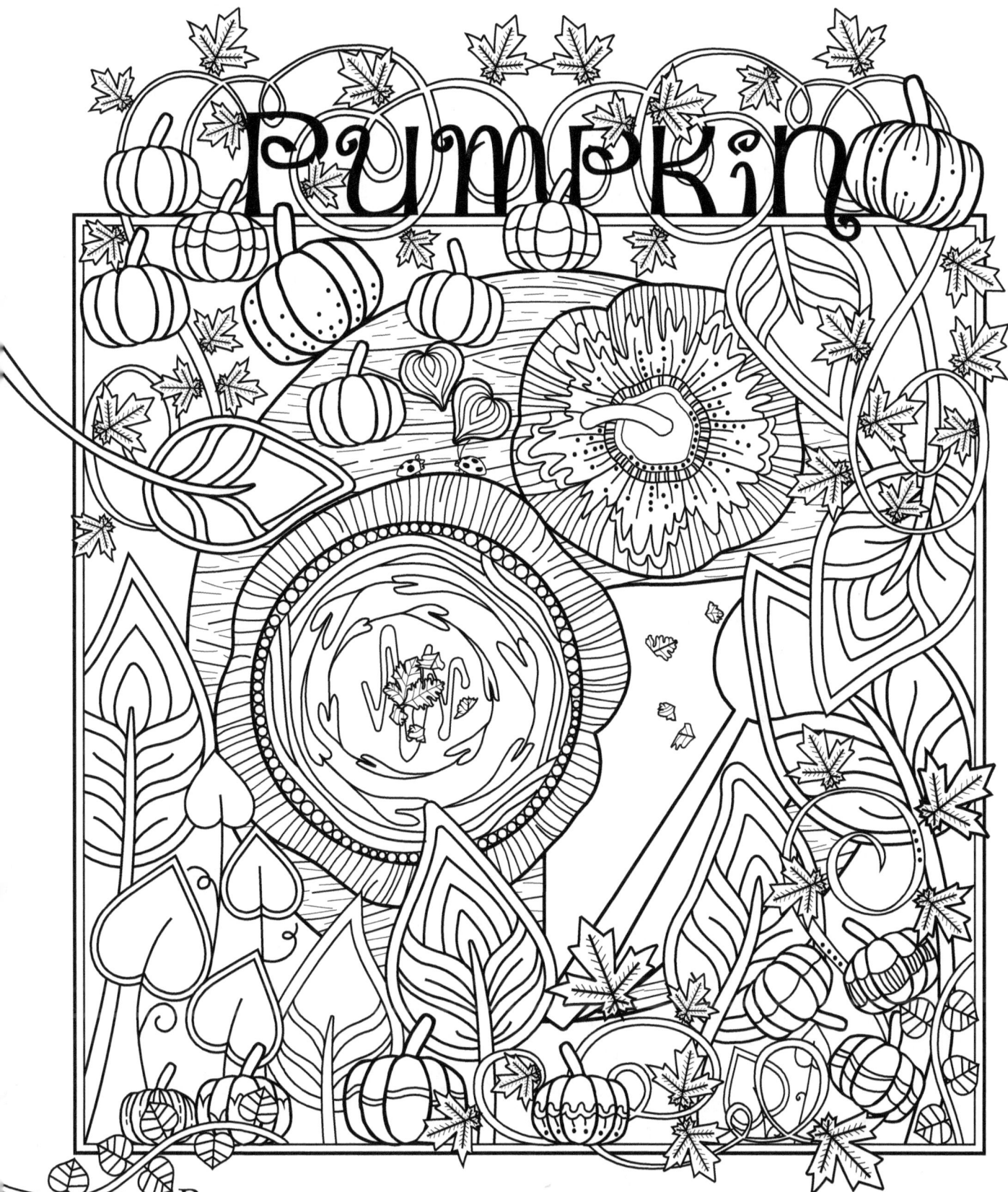

Pumpkin is rich in a variety of vitamins, including; vitamin A, B-complex vitamins, C, E and minerals: iron, manganese, phosphorus and potassium. Pumpkin is rich in the antioxidant beta-carotene (that can convert to vitamin A). Pumpkin contains 3 of the 8 B-complex vitamins: riboflavin (B2), pantothenic acid (B5), and cobalamin (B12). Pumpkin also contains the antioxidant zeaxanthin. Zeaxanthin may protect against age-related vision loss.

PASSIONfruit

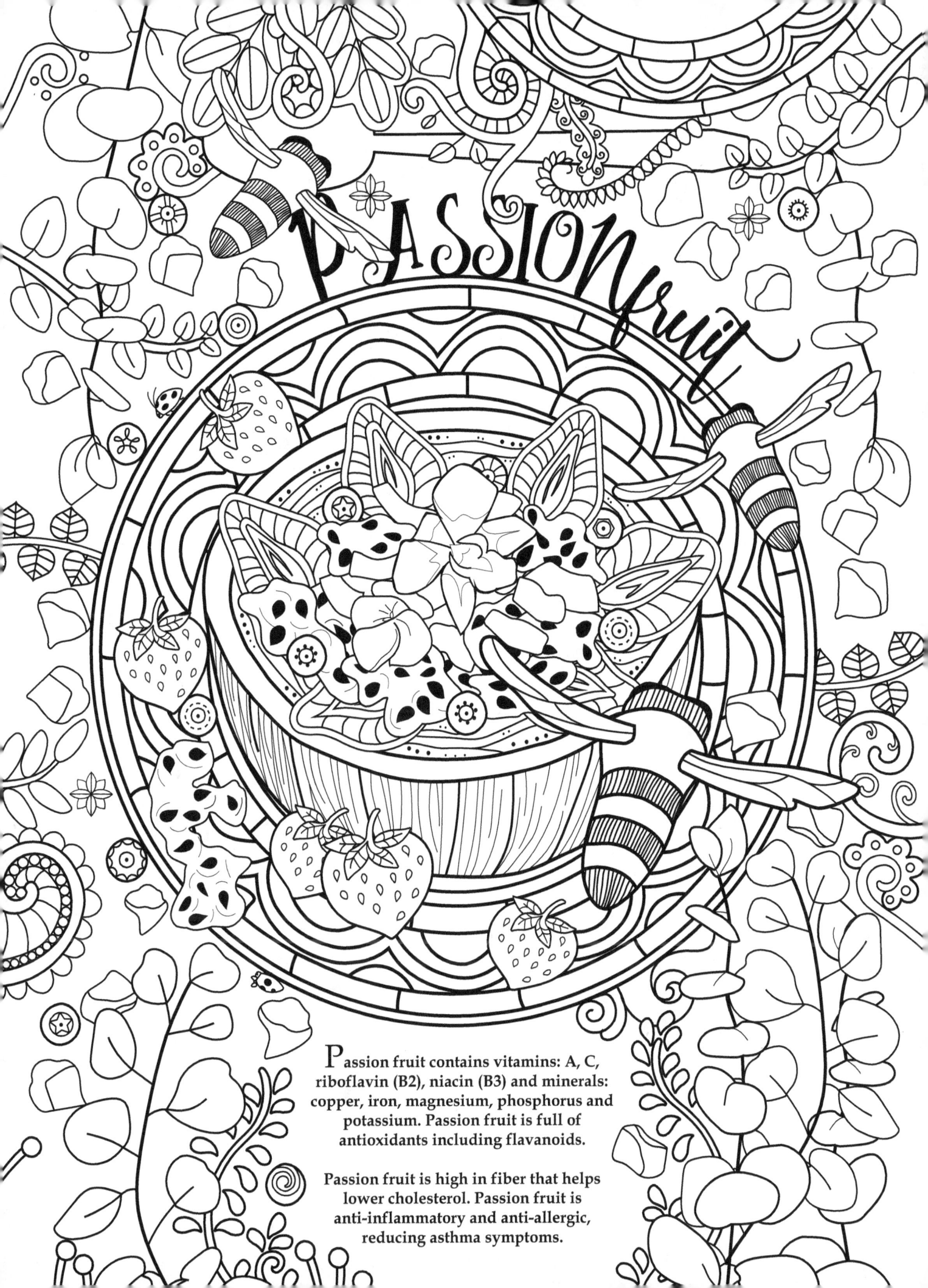

Passion fruit contains vitamins: A, C, riboflavin (B2), niacin (B3) and minerals: copper, iron, magnesium, phosphorus and potassium. Passion fruit is full of antioxidants including flavanoids.

Passion fruit is high in fiber that helps lower cholesterol. Passion fruit is anti-inflammatory and anti-allergic, reducing asthma symptoms.

Legumes

Legumes are the dried fruit of a pod and include: alfalfa sprouts, beans, peanuts and peas! Beans contain vitamins: pyridoxine (B6) and C. B6 is used for energy production, iron absorption and immune function. Beans contain minerals: copper, iron, magnesium, potassium and zinc. Beans are a good source of protein. They are rich in antioxidants and plant compounds including phytosterols that can help to lower cholesterol absorption. Soybeans contain high amounts of isoflavones that are a type of phytoestrogen with estrogenic activity, that mimics human estrogen. Beans may reduce the risk of diabetes, heart disease and certain cancers.

Cruciferous CABBAGE

Cabbage contains vitamin C: thiamin (B1), pyridoxine (B6), folate (B9) and K. Minerals include: calcium, iron, magnesium, manganese, potassium and phosphorus. The apigenin in cabbage (also found in celery and parsley) may help protect against cancer. Anthocyanins – the blue, purple and red pigment found in fruits and vegetables, provides cabbage with beneficial antioxidants.

Cabbage belongs to the cruciferous family of vegetables, that includes; arugula, bok choy, broccoli, brussels sprouts, cauliflower, collard greens and kale. The bitter taste of cruciferous vegetables come from a compound called sulforaphane. Sulforaphane is a potent antioxidant that may have anti-cancer properties. Cruciferous vegetables also contain the plant compound DIM that may protect against the negative effects of radiation.

MINT

Mint contains the highest concentration of antioxidants than any other food. Mint is full of vitamins: beta-carotene (vitamin A), riboflavin (B2), pyridoxine (B6), folate (B9), C, E and K. Minerals include: calcium, iron, magnesium, manganse, and potassium. The Rosmeric Acid in mint may prevent allergies and menthol acts as a decongestant.

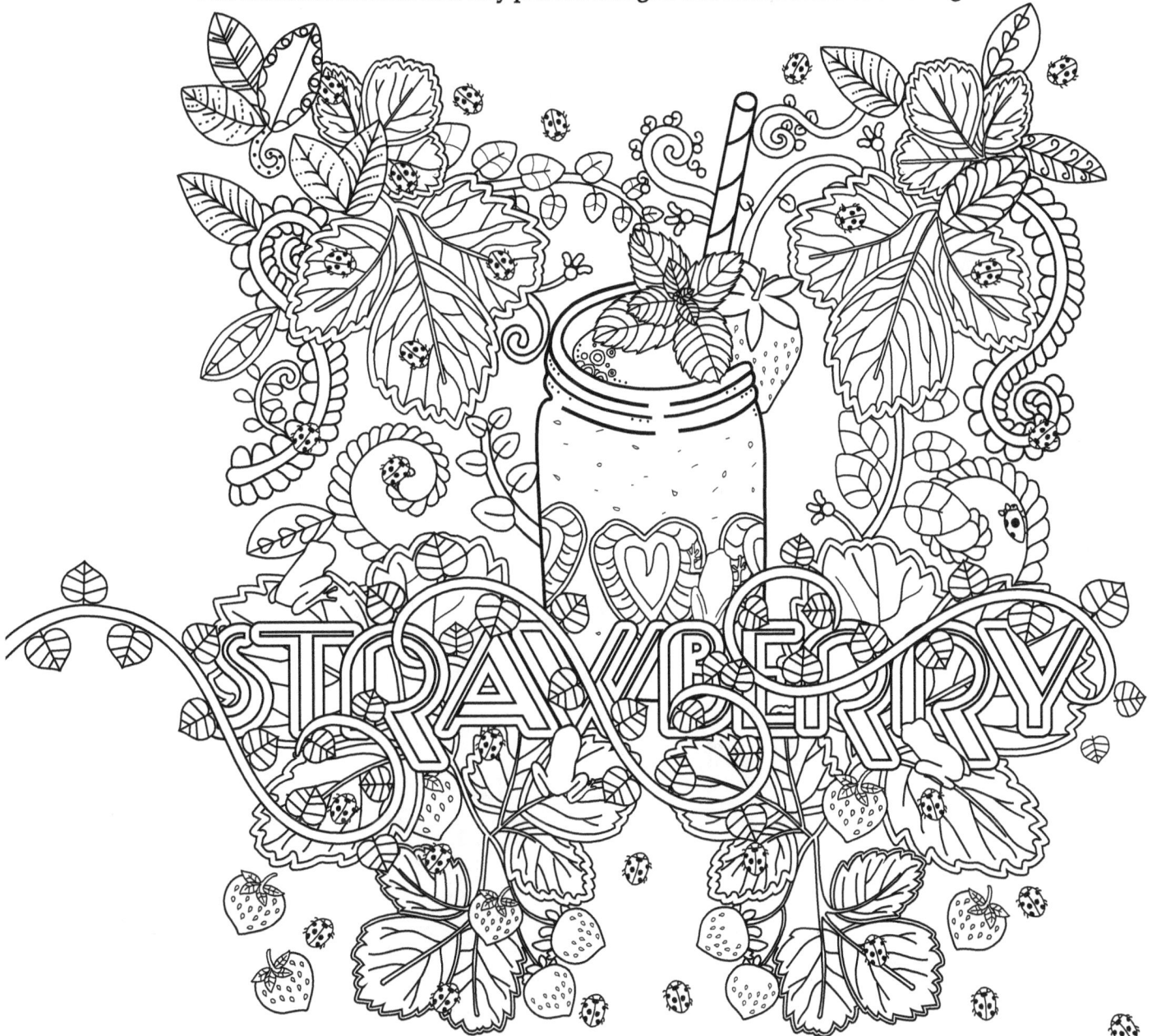

STRAWBERRY

Strawberries contain vitamin C, K, folate (B9), magnesium, manganese and potassium. Strawberries contain anthocyanins, ellagic acid, quercetin and kaempferol that may lower the risk of certain cancers. Strawberries also contain anthocyanins, a flavonoid antioxidant that gives strawberries their red bright color and may help lower the risk of heart disease.

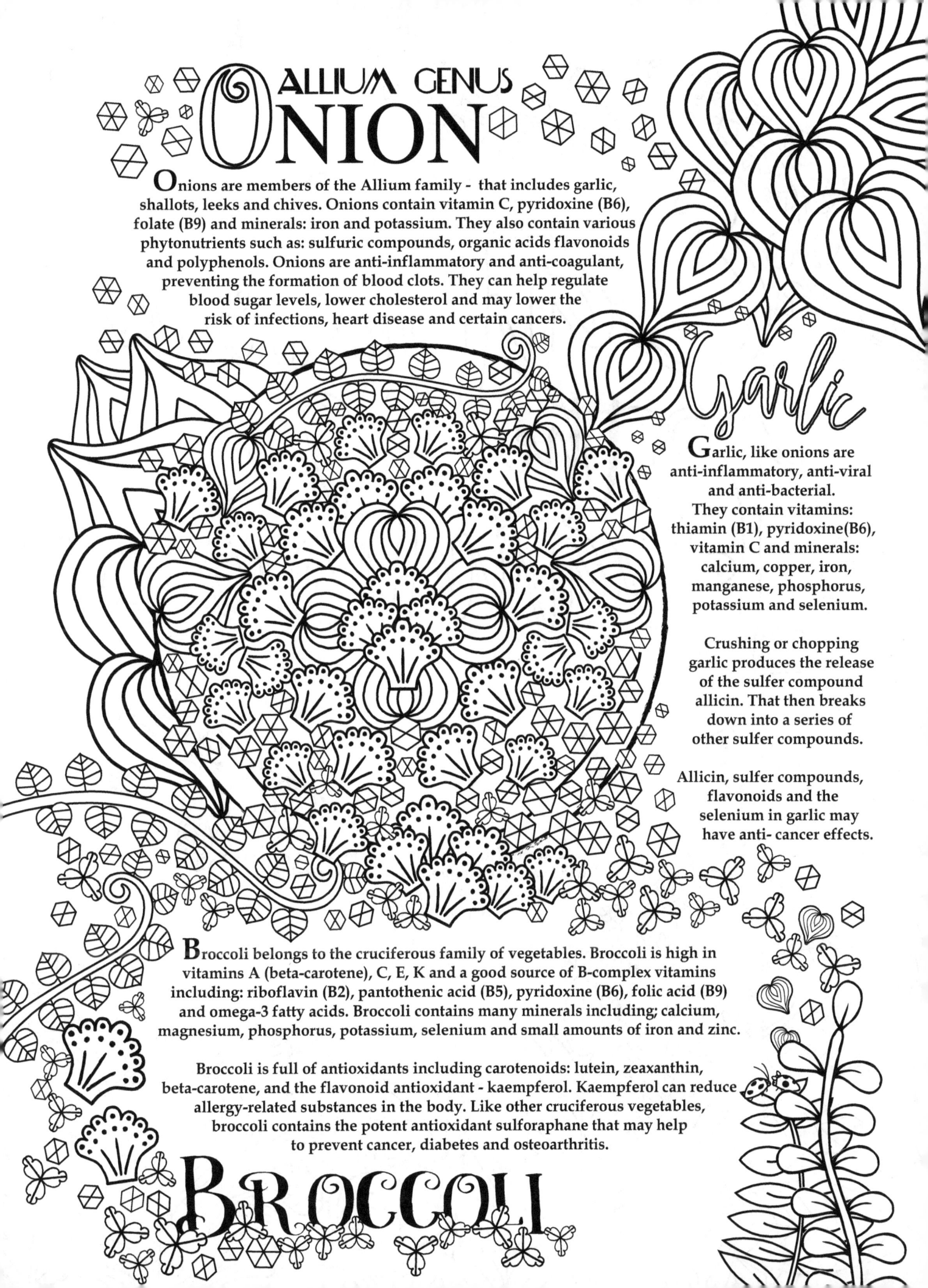

ALLIUM GENUS
ONION

Onions are members of the Allium family - that includes garlic, shallots, leeks and chives. Onions contain vitamin C, pyridoxine (B6), folate (B9) and minerals: iron and potassium. They also contain various phytonutrients such as: sulfuric compounds, organic acids flavonoids and polyphenols. Onions are anti-inflammatory and anti-coagulant, preventing the formation of blood clots. They can help regulate blood sugar levels, lower cholesterol and may lower the risk of infections, heart disease and certain cancers.

Garlic

Garlic, like onions are anti-inflammatory, anti-viral and anti-bacterial. They contain vitamins: thiamin (B1), pyridoxine(B6), vitamin C and minerals: calcium, copper, iron, manganese, phosphorus, potassium and selenium.

Crushing or chopping garlic produces the release of the sulfer compound allicin. That then breaks down into a series of other sulfer compounds.

Allicin, sulfer compounds, flavonoids and the selenium in garlic may have anti- cancer effects.

Broccoli belongs to the cruciferous family of vegetables. Broccoli is high in vitamins A (beta-carotene), C, E, K and a good source of B-complex vitamins including: riboflavin (B2), pantothenic acid (B5), pyridoxine (B6), folic acid (B9) and omega-3 fatty acids. Broccoli contains many minerals including; calcium, magnesium, phosphorus, potassium, selenium and small amounts of iron and zinc.

Broccoli is full of antioxidants including carotenoids: lutein, zeaxanthin, beta-carotene, and the flavonoid antioxidant - kaempferol. Kaempferol can reduce allergy-related substances in the body. Like other cruciferous vegetables, broccoli contains the potent antioxidant sulforaphane that may help to prevent cancer, diabetes and osteoarthritis.

BROCCOLI

Eat from the Rainbow

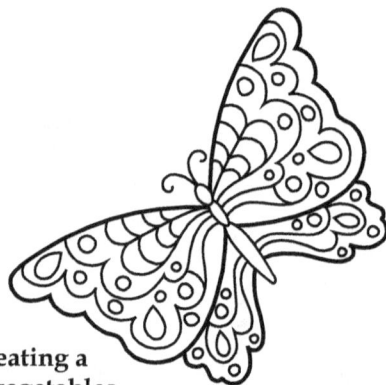

Eat from the rainbow refers to eating a wide variety of colored fruits and vegetables. Ensuring that you get a wide variety of important nutrients.

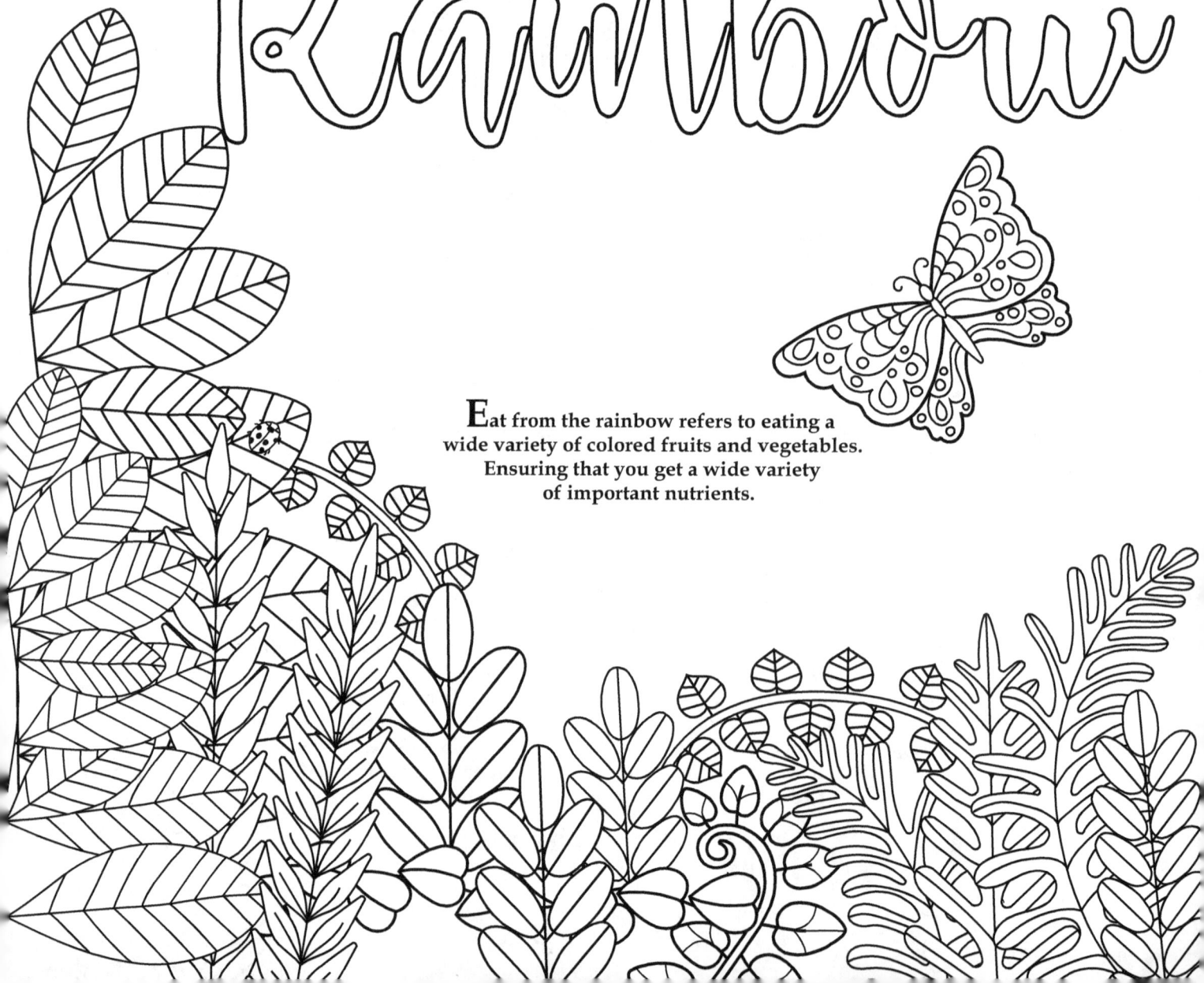

HEALTH NOTES

Vitamins, minerals, essential fatty acids, protien, carbohydrates,
healthy gut bacteria, dietary fiber and many plant compounds
are required for optimal health.

Probiotics, the good gut bacteria also helps aid digestion, support mood and overall health.
Prebiotics, a special form of dietary fiber helps the beneficial probiotic bacteria grow.

Dietary Fiber is important because it helps digestive health,
which is linked to the bodies overall health. Spending short periods of time in the sun
allows your body to absorb vitamin D produced by the skin. Vitamin D may help release
the chemical serotonin, that can also help improve mood.

Healthy eating, fresh air, clean water, rest, exercise and a positive mind set all help
contribute to a healthy body and happy mind.

ABOUT MINERALS

Minerals are important for a healthy body.
There are two types of minerals, major and trace. Major minerals mean
large amounts are required. Trace means small amounts are required.
High levels of minerals can be toxic if over consumed in tablet form.

Major minerals include: calcium, chloride, magnesium,
phosphorous, sodium and sulpher. Trace minerals include: cobalt, copper,
flouride, iodine, iron, maganese, selenium and zinc.
Monitoring iron intake can be important for people eatomg a vegetarian diet.

The Wonderful Wholefood Garden by Karen Martin

Published by HeartAlignBooks

www.thewonderfulwholefoodgarden.com
www.facebook.com/thewonderfulwholefoodfgarden

ISBN: 978-0-646-80100-1

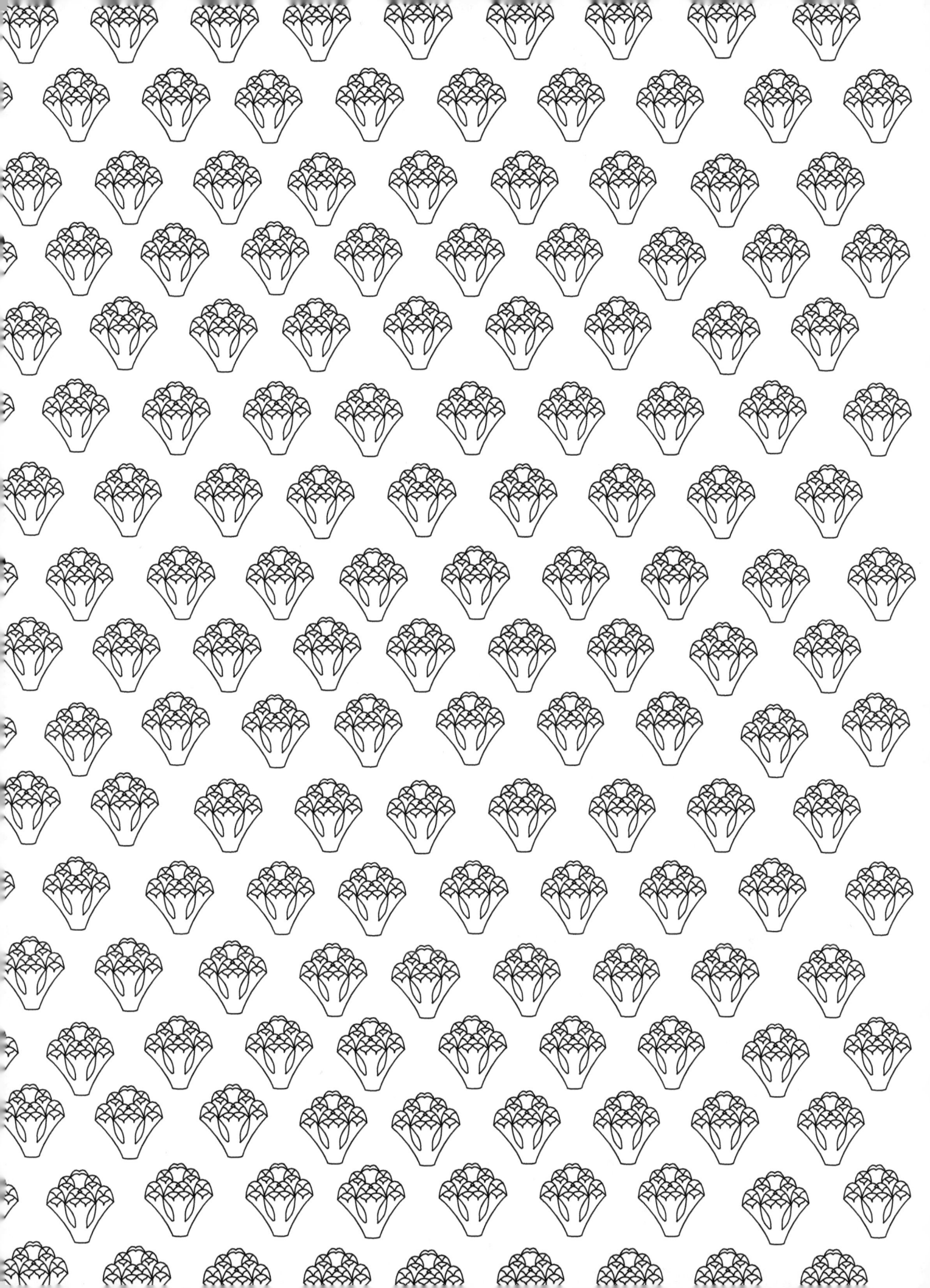

www.ingramcontent.com/pod-product-compliance
Lightning Source LLC
Chambersburg PA
CBHW081410270326
41931CB00016B/3440